SYNOPTIC MEMORIZER OF REPERTORY

Dr. D. G. BAGAL

M.D. (Hom.)

Vice-Principal,

Professor and H.O.D, Department of Repertory

Dr. G. D. Pol Foundation's, Y. M. T. Homoeopathic Medical College,
Navi Mumbai.

Dr. UTTARA AGALE

M.D. (Hom.)

Assistant Professor, Department of Repertory

Dr. G. D. Pol Foundation's, Y. M. T. Homoeopathic Medical College,
Navi Mumbai.

FIRST EDITION

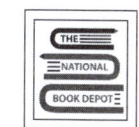

www.nationalbook.com

CBS Publishers & Distributors Pvt Ltd.

First Edition   -   2017

Published by

Raju Shah for

THE NATIONAL BOOK DEPOT

Opp. Wadia Children's Hospital, Parel, Mumbai - 400 012.

Tel : 2416 5274 / 2413 1362 / 24132411 | Fax : 2413 0877

E-mail : nationalbook55@gmail.com

Website : nationalbookdepot.com

and

Satish Kumar Jain for

CBS Publishers & Distributors Pvt Ltd

4819/XI Prahlad Street, 24 Ansari Road, Daryaganj, New Delhi - 110 002, India.

Ph: 23289259, 23266861, 23266867 | Fax: 011-23243014

Website: www.cbspd.com | e-mail: delhi@cbspd.com; cbspubs@airtelmail.in.

Corporate Office: 204 FIE, Industrial Area, Patparganj, Delhi - 110 092.

Ph: 4934 4934 | Fax: 4934 4935 | e-mail: publishing@cbspd.com; publicity@cbspd.com

ISBN : 978-93-80206-83-7

Printed by : Neel Graphics

FOREWORD

It gives me immense pride that Dr. D. G. Bagal and Dr. Uttara Agale made an attempt in publishing the book on Repertory and I happened to write a foreword for it as they are family members of our Dr. G.D. Pol Foundation.

As the book is related to the subject taught by them, it reflects their vast experience in it and the sincere efforts put by them in compiling the book. This type of work requires a lot of concentration and study. I am glad that members from Dr. G. D. Pol Foundation has at least made an attempt to bring it before the profession and thus tries to meet one of the important needs of the profession.

The book has tried to overcome all the lacunas which Undergraduate and Post- graduate students are facing in using repertory. However, it is a continuous process of learning which has made the understanding of book clear and comprehensible for homoeopathic students and practioners. Our authors have magnified the quote by *Benjamin Franklin*: *"Either write something worth reading or do something worth writing".*

I would like to congratulate them and wish them success in their future endeavors.

Hope the subject Repertory is also getting one gem in its crown which will sparkle more than other gems and prove its value in coming days.

Dr. G. D. POL
Chairman
Dr. G. D. Pol Foundationís
Y. M. T. Homoeopathic Medical College
& P. G. Institute, Kharghar, Navi Mumbai.

PREFACE

It is rightly said that *"Necessity is not only the mother of invention, but also the impelling force"* in the preparation of this little book.

A repertory is a place where information is stored or categorized so that it can be retrieved more easily. It is an index of symptoms, with a listing of all of the remedies known to be associated with each particular symptom. The purpose of the repertory is to help you find the right remedy for a given case. It is a tool. The repertory helps to individualize a case to find the right remedy for the right person. It also assists the practitioner find small and rarely used remedies and to link unusual symptoms with the appropriate remedy. There are some cases where using the repertory is crucial to finding the right remedy and other cases where it is much less useful. As it is rightly said by Dr. M. L. Dhawale, *"As repertory is a tool and a tool is best in the hands of a skilled workman and the workman who is not skilled in using repertories naturally blames the tool for unsuccessful results".*

This book is a small and humble attempt to compile the information related with repertories on a single platform. While teaching Undergraduate and Post graduate students it was observed that the students becomes confused due to the vast amount of data and thus makes mistakes and naturally repertory is ignored.

The book incorporates the literature of most commonly used repertories and is more comprehensible for the students in learning and achieving their goals. Synoptic Memorizer of repertory helps to select the correct repertory while repertorizing and will try to eliminate the possible difficulties in using repertories. It is too much to hope that the first edition is entirely free from errors of omission. We are grateful to the readers for the advice if any which will help to improve the subsequent editions of book.

January 2017

Dr. D. G. BAGAL
Dr. UTTARA AGALE

PROLOGUE

An inspirational quote by Brad Henry *"A good teacher can inspire hope, ignite the imagination, and instill a love of learning"*.

The authors have tried to make almost all repertories to study at a glance and it will prove useful to the students as well as to the practitioners. Although there is a vast amount of literature in repertory but it becomes difficult for the beginners to understand the repertory and its gravity. So, many a times students develop less interest in repertory and many times those who fail in making the repertory techniques useful again blames the repertory.

But this book is a sincere effort in making the study of repertory more simpler and easier for the students and beginners. It was the need of time to assemble the information in a systematic and organized way and "Synoptic Memorizer of Repertory" has proved it.

As it is said by Todd Park *"Data by itself is useless. Data is only useful if you apply it"*.

The book starts with the introduction on case taking and introduction of repertory which is further followed by all different types of repertories with their philosophies and plan and constructions. There are distinguishing points which make the concept clear of students while learning. The hard work of authors is reflected in this book for which I want to mention a saying by C. S. Lewis that "Hardships often prepare ordinary people for an extraordinary destiny".

As this book is an attempt so in subsequent years it will become masterpiece in the subject. I would like to congratulate them and wish them success in their future endeavors

Dr. ARUN BHASME
VICE-PRESIDENT
C. C. H. NEW DELHI.

DEDICATED

IN THE MEMORY OF MY

FATHER

Late. Mr. GOVIND MADHAV BAGAL

(1925-1995)

WITH HIS BLESSINGS AND TEACHINGS

MY LIFE FLOURISHED

AND

TO THOSE WHO LOVE

AND WORK FOR REPERTORY

ACKNOWLEDGEMENT

We would like thank Dr. (Mrs.) P. P. Page, Principal of Dr. G. D. Pol Foundation's Y. M. T. Homoeopathic Medical College, Kharghar, Navi Mumbai for being constant inspiration for us and Dr. Ravi Bhosale Principal, Sawkar, Homoeopathic Medical College, Satara for his support.

We would like to thank our family members for staying with us in all thick and thin and giving strength to us.

Last but not least we would like to express our gratitude to all the teaching and non-teaching staff of Dr. G. D. Pol Foundation's Y. M. T. Homoeopathic Medical College, Kharghar, Navi Mumbai for their support.

Dr. D. G. BAGAL
Dr. UTTARA AGALE

CONTENT

SECTION I

SECTION II

SECTION III

Repertories

SECTION I

A. INTRODUCTION

Definition

A case is not merely a collection of symptoms, but it comprises totality of disease, a change in the whole person from the state of health to the state of sickness. It constitutes expressions from mental and physical plane.

H. A. Robert has said – The combination of subjective and objective symptoms comprise the case.

The foremost step towards making a good prescription is a well taken case.

HAHNEMANN writes

"If the physician clearly perceives what is to be cured in disease, that is to say, in every individual case of disease (*knowledge of disease*, indications), if he clearly perceives what is curative in medicines, that is to say in each individuals medicine (*knowledge of medical powers*), and if he knows how to adapt, according to clearly defined principles, what is curative in medicines to what he has discovered to be undoubtedly morbid in the patient, so that the recovery must ensure-to adapt it, as well in respect to the suitability of the medicine most appropriate according to its mode of action to the case before him (choice of the remedy, the medicine indicated), as also in respect to the exact mode of preparation and quantity of it required (proper dose), and the proper period for repeating the dose; if finally, he knows the obstacles to recovery in each case and is aware how to remove them, so that the restoration may be permanent: then he understands how to treat judiciously & rationally, and he is a true practitioner of the healing art"...........................

Para – 3 of **Organon of Medicine**

Case taking is an art on which the success or failure depends.

A proper case taking is essential for the success process of the study of the Repertory and repertorization. Further, the art of the physician in taking the case must so record it that we may glean from this record those elements that may be translated into the rubrics of the repertory. However, it is impossible to secure from the patient a clear-cut picture of his difficulties, in spite of the best art the physician may exercise.

Talking to the patients and obtaining their health histories are usually the first and often the most important parts of the health case process.

OBJECTIVES OF CASE TAKING:

1) To diagnose the disease and case.

2) To understand the person as a whole from its social, interpersonal sectors.

3) Collection of all the facts pertaining to the patient, which may help in reaching to the totality of the patient and thereby help in finding the correct similimum.

4) To manage the case-auxiliary, general and specific.

B. DIRECTIONS OF CASE TAKING

Approach to the Patient

The physician should approach his patients with humility and gratitude, with confidence and pride in the responsibility which will be his for the remainder of his life. It is all a matter of communication between patient and physician. It is no exaggeration to say that even facial expression, tone of voice and manner of movement can affect the ability to elicit the patient's story and to lead him back to health. For it is in such outward signs that we display those attitudes of mind – impatience, boredom, embarrassment, disbelief and reproach – which act as barrier to communication with others. In the presence of his patients, the physician must master his emotions, clear his mind of distracting thoughts and avoid all appearances of haste. His manner should be alert and attentive yet gentle and sympathetic. Without these qualities, he will neither obtain the facts needed for the diagnosis nor effectively convey the advice essential to the patient.

The Disease…

Disease is a departure from health and is manifested in an individual during life by symptoms. These symptoms are as under:

- **Subjective Symptoms** are those symptoms that are recognizable only by the patient and present no external indications such as pain, itching or a feeling of chilliness etc. Philosophically Subjective reality that exists in the mind only!

- **Objective Symptoms** are those that can be detected by observer e.g. abdominal enlargement or dullness on percussion. Philosophically objective reality is that which can be demonstrated by means of tangible or outward signs, good deal of pain.

The word symptom is used in two senses. Sometime it used in a general sense to indicate all the subjective & objective evidence of a disease; but more usually it is employed in a narrow sense, as synonymous with subjective symptoms. Objective symptoms are usually spoken of as signs; and those objective symptoms, which are made out by physical examination, are known as physical signs.

Just as the value and significance of physical signs depend on the skill and experience of the physician who observes them, so the significance of subjective symptoms has to be weighed and considered in relation to the character and constitution of the patient who complains of them. Thus a certain symptom may appear trivial and unimportant to a patient of strong character not addicted to introspection, although serious disease may be present; whereas in women with a susceptible nervous system every subjective symptom, however slight, may cause great anxiety, exaggeration, and even real suffering. Sub-mammary pain, for instance, in the first might indicate aneurysm; in the second, hysteria.

- **General (or constitutional) symptoms** are those, which relate to the whole body, such as debility or pyrexia.

Hahnemann writes (Para 71 Organon of Medicine) "As it is now no longer a matter of doubt that the diseases of mankind consist merely of groups of certain symptoms and of mankind and transformed into health by medicinal substances but only by such as are capable of artificially producing morbid symptoms (and such is the process in all genuine cures), hence the operation of curing is comprised in the following points":

- How is the physician to ascertain what is necessary to be known in order to cure the disease? (Case Taking)
- How is he to gain knowledge of the instruments adapted for the cure of the natural disease, the pathogenetic powers of the medicines?
- What is the most suitable method of employing these artificial morbific agents (medicines) for the cure of natural disease?

In case taking, our objective is, first, to elicit all the data of the case; and, secondly, by reasoning based on those data to arrive at its Diagnosis, Prognosis and Treatment. It will be found in actual practice that everything turns on the diagnosis; this is our first and principal object; the prognosis and treatment follow from this.

The investigation of a case consists of four parts:

A) The Interrogation of the Patient
B) The Physical Examination
C) The special investigation
   Ancillary Methods (e.g., Radiology, Clinical Pathology), where necessary
D) Interrogation of relatives and friends.

A. **Interrogation of the Patient: By interrogating the patient the objective is to obtain the following information:**

- What is his/her chief or cardinal symptom?
- The facts concerning the present illness,
- The patient's previous history,
- The patient's personal history, and
- His/her family history

Throughout the interrogation of the patient it is well to follow three general rules:

1. **Avoid putting "leading questions"** i.e., questions that suggest their own answer: e.g., "Have you had a pain in the back?" suggests an obvious answer to the patient. It might be put thus: "Have you had any pain, and if so, where?" The patient should be encouraged to tell his own story, without interruption. Moreover, the very words he uses should be recorded between inverted commas, and on no account should his words be translated into scientific terms. Some say that leading questions are permissible when the patient is very ignorant and stupid, but these are the very cases in which leading questions should be specially avoided. The only legitimate way of putting a leading question is in an alternative form – e.g., "Have you suffered from diarrhea or constipation?" Time, patience and tact are necessary to elicit the true facts of the case, without irrelevant detail. Our object is to learn what the patient feels and knows, not what he thinks of his disease; and our patience is often sorely tried by a long story of his own or his previous doctors' views on his case.

Our record should be comprehensive, including all-important data, negative as well as positive, yet concise i.e., excluding irrelevant facts. Only experience and knowledge of medicine can teach us what is or is not relevant. The beginner should strive after completeness rather than conciseness.

2. **A chronological order should always be adopted,**

both in eliciting and in recording the facts. Nothing is more wearisome than to wade through a mass of verbiage, which mixes up dates. Dates should be recorded always in the same terms. It is very common, for instance, to read in students' reports that "breathlessness began in the year 1952", "palpitation started when the patient was aged forty," "edema came on two years ago".

3. **Always adopt a kindly and sympathetic manner**.

Not only is it our bounden duty to be considerate and patient with those who suffer, but by entering into the spirit of the patient's sufferings we can often get at more important facts, and a truer narration of them, than can one whose harsh or abrupt manner causes the patient to shrink up like an oyster into its shell. Put your question s in as simple and non-technical a form as possible, and be sure that the patient attaches the same meaning to the words as you do. Much will depend on the tact of the physician, and two very good rules may here be added – viz., Never enquire concerning a family history of a lethal illness such as cancer before a patient whose illness is likely to be of that nature; Never put questions bearing on venereal disease before the husband or wife of the patient.

a. **The Chief or Cardinal Symptom** : The first question to ask a patient should always be the same "What do you complain of?" Special attention should be paid to the main symptom for which the patient seeks advice or is admitted to hospital, because it is this symptom, which guides most of our subsequent inquiries. It should always, as far as possible, be recorded in the patient' s own words. The best way to avoid error is to verify your observations by repeating your examination.

b. **The History of the Present Illness** must be taken and recorded with care. Some patients come out at once with their story; others remain silent. The former must not be interrupted except to steer them away from irrelevancy. The latter should be gently encouraged rather than questioned. In other words, the patient's history should whenever possible be received, not taken.

Most patients expect the doctor to make the first move. After a few words to put the patient at ease, he must find out why the patient has come. The conventional opening question "What do you complain of?" is not always suitable. Some patients have no real symptoms but feel obliged to mention a minor discomfort in answer to this question when in fact they have come with a problem rather than a pain. The more sympathetic question, "What can I do to help you?" sometimes brings a more revealing answer. However, more than one approach may have to be made before the appropriate response is obtained; a list of suggested alternative is given as under: Whether the patient is presenting with a symptom or a problem, this should be recorded in the patient's own words, along with note of its duration. If the patient's own words consist of a diagnosis rather than a symptom, he must be asked to indicate how this condition affects him. The symptoms and not the "diagnosis" are then recorded e.g. Chest pain: One week, Cough: 2 moths etc.

Questionnaire
- What do you feel wrong with yourself?
- In what way do you feel ill?
- What can I do to help you?
- Tell me why you wanted to have homoeopathic treatment?

When the patient is finished his story and answered "No" to the question: "Have you any other symptom at all?", he may then be asked leading questions to ensure that no symptom has been forgotten.

Onset (record for each symptom in chronological order)
- When did you (symptom) first start?
- Were you perfectly well before then?
- Have you ever had anything like this before?
- Did your (symptom) come suddenly one day or gradually

  or periodically?
- What were you doing when it came on? (if onset is sudden)
  Development (record for each symptom in chronological order)

- What has happened to your (symptom) since then?
- Coming & going? (record frequency, duration & relationship if any to physiological or environmental factors) Getting worse or better? (Record whether the change has been gradual; if not, then when it occurred and whether related to physiological or environmental factors. Description (pain given here as an example)
- Show me where you feel pain?
- Does it move anywhere?
- What kind of pain is it? (aching, stabbing, throbbing, gripping etc)
- How bad is it? Does it make you stop what you are doing?
- How often do you get it? (record whether continues or number of times per day, week, month or year)
- How long does it last?
- Does it come at any special time?
- Does anything bring it on or make it worse?
- Does anything relieve it? What do you do when it comes out?
- Do you feel anything else wrong at the same time?

It cannot too strongly be emphasized that in many diseases a full and accurate history of the illness may be the only method of arriving at a diagnosis, for physical signs may be absent or in abeyance (e.g., in angina pectoris). Taking an average, it is fair to compute that of the in formation on which a diagnosis is ultimately founded, at least 50 per cent comes from an accurate history, and rather less than 50 per cent, from the physical examination and subsequent special investigations. The history should then reveal:

i. The mode of onset, whether sudden or gradual,

ii. What the patient was doing at the time, and whether he attributed the onset to any cause. In many cases it is necessary to enquire into

iii. Whether the symptom is localized or widespread,

iv. Does it radiate to other areas; also

v. The duration of the symptom,

vi. Whether it ended suddenly or gradually,

vii. Its severity,

viii. Whether it has occurred since, and if so, how many times, and is it getting more or less severe,

ix. What intervals of freedom have occurred, when the patient has been entirely free of the symptom,

x. Have other symptoms occurred in association with this chief symptom, and if so, what are they,

xi. What does the patient do during the time of the symptom to relieve it,

xii. Has the patient found any measures of avail to ward off attacks, e.g., drugs, diet, etc. In many cases, e.g., in juvenile and unconscious persons, the history has to be elicited from near relatives or friends. It is useful also to know whether the patient has recently been, or is now, under medical care, not only because the symptoms may have been modified by treatment, but also because one of the most important ethical principles of the medical profession may be involved. In all these enquiries the above stated general rules given above apply.

c. **The Previous History** of the patient bears largely on the etiology, or causation, of his illness, and deals with any illnesses the patient may have had. Note in chronological order all ailments from which the patient has suffered prior to the present one, with the dates of their occurrence and their duration: e.g., contagious diseases of childhood; and especially previous operations or serious illnesses. If the illnesses have been at all obscure, it is desirable to add a few of the leading symptoms to prove the nature of the alleged attacks, and in such instances inverted commas should be freely used. For instance "rheumatism" is vague terms which may mean any disease attended by pains in the limbs, such as are due to alcoholism, syphilis, tabes dorsalis or neurasthenia. The subject of syphilis should always be approached with delicacy in the case of women. Indirect information may often be gained by enquiring for prolonged sore throat, followed by loss of hair, enlarged glands, skin rashes, etc. In married women, a series of stillbirths, or children born with eruptions or snuffles, may have the same significance.

Questionnaire
- Have you had any serious illness in the past?
- How did it affect you?
- Any operation or bad injuries?
- Any stillbirth, miscarriage or problem in pregnancy?
- Have you ever been to hospital?
- Have you missed time from work because of illness?

- Have you ever visited doctor before?
- Have you ever had (here list illness possibly relevant to present complaint)

d. **The Personal History** must be enquired into such as:

    i. Present and previous occupations;

    ii. Previous residence abroad;

    iii. The home conditions;

    iv. Habits as to alcohol and tobacco and whether alcohol (e.g., wine, beer or spirits) is taken between or with meals, because more harm is done by alcohol before meals (especially cocktails) than many times the same quantity taken with meals;

    v. The appetite;

    vi. The state of the digestion and the bowels;

    vii. The weight, and whether this is constant, being gained or lost;

    viii. The general state of the nervous system, e.g., depression, excitability, nervousness;

    ix. The orientation of the patient to his (or her) work and to home life, and whether there are any special anxieties attached to these;

    x. The amount and quality of sleep;

    xi. In women, the previous state of the catamenia, and the number of pregnancies, miscarriages or stillbirths, should be noted.

e. **The Family History** may, like the previous history, have a casual relationship to the patient's illness. The age and state of health if living, age and cause of death if dead, of near relations, should always be noted: i.e., father and mother, brothers and sisters, sons and daughters, also of husband or wife. Enquiry should also be made as to whether any members of the family (parents, grandparents, brothers, sisters, uncles, aunts or cousins) have suffered from tuberculosis, cancer, acute rheumatism, gout, nervous disease, asthma, heart disease, apoplexy, and especially those diseases to which the patient himself seems liable.

Questionnaire

- Are you married?
- Is your wife/husband well?
- Do you have children? (record age & sex)
- Have they ever been seriously ill (record details)
- Have you lost any children? (record age & cause of death)
- Do you have brothers & sisters (record age & sex)
- Have they ever been seriously ill? (record details)
- Have you lost any brothers or sisters? (record age & cause of death)
- Are both of your parents living? (if not, give age & cause of death)
- Have they ever been seriously ill? (record details)
- Do you know of any one in the family with symptoms like yours?
- Do you know of any disease affecting more than one member of your family?

f. **Social History**, question asked under this heading are designed to uncover anything in the patient's personal life, relevant to either the cause or management of his ill health. We need therefore, to know about his work, hobbies, habits, environment at home, visits abroad, domestic and marital life any potential source of mental illness.

Questionnaire

- Are you working?
- What exactly do you do? (record hours, physical activity, potential hazards, traveling)
- How long you have done this job?
- What jobs have you done before, starting when you left school? (record as above)
- What do you do in your spare time? (hobbies, sports etc.)
- Are your mealtimes regulars?
- When is your main meal?
- Do you or did you smoke? (record duration, number of cigarettes/cigars/pipes per day)
- Do you or did you take alcohol? (record type & amount)
- Do you or did you take drugs of any kind? (record type & amount)
- Have you been abroad? (record where & when)
- Tell me about your home? (rooms, stairs, toilet facilities, state of repair)
- Who is living in the same house?
- Have any been ill recently?
- Do you have animals at home?
- Have you had any recent worries or stresses?

B. Physical Examination:

1. Here, again, having learned by interrogation our patient's chief complaint, we should ask ourselves, is there any striking or predominant sign or appearance? The importance of inspecting our patient cannot be overestimated. In these days of scientific instruments we are too likely to forget to use our own faculties. By simply using our eyes many important data may be learned besides the color of the skin, the condition of the teeth and gums, the general nutrition, the attitude or decubitus, and the facial expression. For instance, the manner in which a patient answers questions is often the first clue to anxiety, and a peculiar mode of speech is one of the pathognomonic signs of general paralysis of the insane, disseminated sclerosis and other diseases. Moreover, with experience we can by this means form a conclusion as to the kind of patient we have to deal with. Again, never be in a hurry; only by taking time can we fully appreciate all the points presented to us. This habit of "observing" the patient is only developed by long practice; it will never be developed if the young physician allows himself to be infected by the hurry of modern times.

2. It is important always to commence examination with that **ORGAN TO WHICH THE SYMPTOMS ARE MAINLY REFERABLE.** Some teachers direct their pupils, to examine and report on the physiological systems always in the same order (first the heart, then the lungs, then the digestive system and so forth), whatever, may be the illness.

But such a course has three objections:

i. The student goes about his work in a mechanical fashion;

ii.   If the patient suffers from some serious disorder, such as peritonitis, he may be exhausted by a complete investigation of the chest and other parts during the acute illness; and

iii. Often it is a waste of time to examine all the organs with equal thoroughness. The same educational advantages and experience can be obtained by the other method, and in th at way we come to the most important facts first.

3.   In all cases **EVERY ORGAN IN THE BODY SHOULD BE CAREFULLY EXAMINED;** for although we may find in one physiological system sufficient mischief to account for the patient's symptoms, the other organs may reveal changes, which considerably modify treatment, prognosis & even diagnosis. Whatever order is adapted; the student should not wander from organ to organ, but examine each physiological system thoroughly before proceeding to the next.

It is best to get in to the habit of adopting some such order of physical examination as the following: first, note the general conditions; second, examine the organ chiefly affected; third, other organs in the following order: Thorax (heart and lungs), Abdomen (alimentary canal, liver, spleen and genito-urinary system), Head and Limbs (nervous and motor systems).

The examination should always be carried out gently and without undue exposure. In serious cases, especially when the heart or lungs are involved, it is often well to postpone a thorough examination of some organs, so as not to risk harming the patient by exposing or fatiguing him. On the other hand,

the young physician should never allow modesty to prevent his making a through decision. This rule is more necessary in sensitive patients, but a little firmness, tact, and a courteous demeanor will generally enable him to perform what is a duty both to his patient and to himself.

After completing the above schedule, we have to individualize remedies and patient. The concept of individualization as reflected in the totality of the symptoms furnishes the only sound basis for selection of remedy in Homoeopathy practice. Individualization is another name for a process of synthesis done after the analysis of an accurate and complete data recorded after observation and examination of the patient.

As individuality of each man is unique, his reactions to environment and other factors also vary from man to man. In homoeopathic language such a concept of a whole and an individual man that is ill, is expressed through "totality of symptoms" which is indicative of the deviation from the total state of health.

In homoeopathy the entire examination of a patient is conducted with a view to discovering not only the general or common features of the case by which it is classified diagnostically and pathologically, but also the special and particular symptoms which differentiate the case from others of the same general class. It recognizes the fact that no two cases or patients, even with the same disease are exactly alike. In actual practice the "differences" are very often the deciding factor in the choice of the remedy.

Homeopathically each symptom of the patient's sickness has to be modified by the following factors before going for Repertorisation/Simllimum:

- Laterality or sides
- Time-hour
- Modifications-conditions, circumstances
- Extension
- Location
- Character or kind of sensation

In **Organon para 83-104**, Hahnemann provides the complete instructions for "Case taking". ACCORDING **TO THE MASTERS, MOST HOMOEOPATHIC DOCTORS MAKE THE THREE MISTAKES IN CASE TAKING**

- **Interruption**
- **Yes or No answers**
- **Confirming the remedy you want (Pet remedy)**

HAHNEMANN writes

"…..he then makes a note of what he himself observes in the patient and ascertains how much of that peculiar to the patient in his healthy state" **(para 90 of Organon).**

How to Diagnose?

It is always important that how the data elicited may be utilized in order to arrive at Diagnosis. An attempt is made to find a single diagnosis which will account for most or all the facts of the case. If some facts do not fit the pattern appropriate to diagnoses, their accuracy must be checked and the original diagnosis reviewed before two or more separate diagnosis are postulated. A complete diagnosis would describe the patient's illness in terms of the site (Anatomy: where?), nature (Pathophysiology: what?) and cause (Etiology: why?) of the disease process. In most instances, however, the physician has to satisfied with a differential diagnosis which admits to more that a single possible answer to one or more of these questions. The alternative diagnosis should be listed in order of probability and reasons given in support of the one which is preferred.

When considering the differential diagnosis, priority must always be given to the problems for which the patient sort medical advise.

C. Special Investigations:

Having arrived at a tentative diagnosis, it is always advisable to confirm (where ever applicable) this by the use of X-rays, pathological tests, and other special methods of investigations. These should only be used in confirmation of a clinical diagnosis and should never replace the interrogation and physical examination of the patient in the search for a diagnosis.

D. Interrogation of relatives and friends.

The symptoms which remain unnoticed by the physician and overlooked by the patient himself are best narrated by the relatives and friends. The details about which the physician don't want to rely on patient can be cross examined with the relatives and friends.

In cases of poisonings and accidents the history can be asked from the relatives and friends who were present at the site or who are close to the patient.

C. CASE RECEIVING AND DESIRED QUALITIES OF PHYSICIAN

Individualization forms one of the most important pillars, on which stands the portal of Homeopathy. A physician cannot think of prescribing unless he has learned the art of deducing uncommon from the common mass. This can only be attained when he judiciously receives the whole case and henceforth moves towards extracting of characteristics from it. Receiving of Case, as it may seem to a layman is not an easy task. It is acquired through years of persistent labor and experience.

So, can just obtaining the knowledge, reading books make one adept in this art? It is not so, it requires qualities of mind and soul which makes one an expert in this art.

> "The individualizing examination of a case of disease, for which I shall only give in this place general directions, of which the practitioner will bear in mind only what is applicable for each individual case, demands of the physician nothing but freedom from prejudice and sound senses, attention in observing and fidelity in tracing the picture of the disease".

In this aphorism Hahnemann has given the motive, requisites and method of case taking. The sole motive of case taking is **"formulating the image of the sick"** through the bringing out the individualizing features of the case.

Now we see for case taking:

Purpose = Formulating the image of the sick

Methodology = Bringing out the individualizing features of the sick

Requirements = Freedom from prejudice and Sound senses

Attentive Observing mind

Fidelity in tracing the picture of the disease

In the above aphorism (83), Hahnemann asserts the desired qualifications in a physician. He is so particular about these as he believed that only a proper physician (who has all the requisites) would be able to imbibe and practice his directions in dealing with different cases, in different ways according to the circumstances, which he plans to explain in the later Aphorisms (84-99).

Freedom from prejudice Hahnemann had already discussed about the qualities of a physician and about his knowledge in previous aphorisms e.g. Aph. 6 and 3. As per the quality is concerned he said that the physician should be unprejudiced and as per the knowledge he said that the physician should have detailed knowledge about what is to be cured in the disease and what is curable in medicine i.e. he should have the knowledge of the disease process and the knowledge of the medicine.

Now why he again refers to the word "freedom from prejudiced" before explaining the case receiving guidelines? This is so because he wants to remind us that every physician has to know with their sound senses that which aphorism will be applicable to the given case and which aphorism will not be applicable, without being prejudiced. It is essential to testify through all aphorisms and ascertain that to which aphorism the case belongs. This can be understand by the following examples.

A person often exaggerates his symptoms to draw the attention of the physician; this does not mean that we take the Rubric *crying pain with or pain agonizing*. We should have the freedom of mind and use our sound senses to discriminate whether the patient's agony is due to pain or only he is doing it to impress the physician and should be listed under Hypochondriac patient mentioned in Aph. 98.

Now the guideline and the plan of treatment to deal with this kind of cases will be different if we do not have the freedom of mind and we can select the rubric crying pain with which actually does not belong to the patient and can lead to the wrong section of medicine.

So Hahnemann teaches us to be free from prejudice and have sound senses to use his guidelines whenever needed.

Attentive Observing mind:

To observe means to look without judgement, to witness without analysis.

Attentive means giving close and thoughtful attention.

> Necessity of attentive observing mind is explained by the Hahnemann in Aphorism 84 as he describes *"The patient details the history of his sufferings; those about him tell what they heard him complain of, how he has behaved and what they have noticed in him; the physician sees, hears, and remarks by his other senses ..."*

This means that all our senses, including our awareness and observation and the inner senses have to be concentrated towards patient at the time of case receiving. We have to be completely observant; we need to focus our senses, attention and observation towards patient.

Fidelity in tracing the picture of the disease: Fidelity means faithfulness. Here Hahnemann wants the physician to be faithful in drawing the picture of the sick. One must pay faithful attention on the symptoms narrated by the patient, the behavior of the patient and the observations made by the attendants and physician himself. After this he should use his common senses to arrange the data given by the patient and process it to decide the further plan of treatment.

D. ANALYSIS OF CASE FOR REPERTORIZATION

The word Analysis originates from the Greek word, *analusis* meaning "breaking up or dissolving". Its literal meaning is the process of breaking up of a complex topic into constitutional parts to gain a better understanding of the subject. This method of systematic study has long been used by *Descartes, Galileo, Newton* as a practical method of physical discovery.

According to Dr. Castro, "The act of resolving or reducing or breaking the whole into pieces or groups is called analysis".

Analysis of Symptoms is important for homeopaths as it helps us in understanding the case. We understand health and disease as a Gestalt concept and not just the haphazard conglomeration of symptoms. The study of constituents and their inter-relationships help us in understanding the concept of "WHOLE" - a vital aspect in the understanding of homeopathy.

After a thorough case taking a physician is in possession of a large number of symptoms which if selected and arranged properly could help in forming a complete picture of the case. Also it includes the most important task of assessing the relative value of each part of the case alone and in relation to the whole. Therefore, Analysis of Case is the logical dismemberment of the case recorded into viable units which help in perfect synthesis. This process is not mechanical but an artistic pursuit with a logical mind. It is like extracting of 24 carat gold from its ore; a sort of carving out the perfect sculpture of Madonna from the large marble block.

But, yes it needs the art and expertise of Michelangelo.

Proper analysis needs a keen and analytical mind. The physician should be able to analyze every symptom in depth and to arrange it logically. The physician is required to be unprejudiced, observant of details and with analytical approach.

But as important it may seem it is the step where one very frequently errs. A slight error on the part of physician can mislead the whole case leading to improper selection of medicine. As it all depends on his discretion alone about the separation and arrangement of each symptom which help in synthesizing the complete picture.

Different stalwarts with different philosophies have their views about analyzing of case but the underlying theory remains the same.

Hahnemannian Viewpoint : Dr. Hahnemann in his Organon stated the importance of characteristic symptom. According to him a case presents with symptoms, most of which are general and undefined whereas some are *more striking, singular, uncommon and peculiar* (characteristic). It is these characteristics which are given higher priority while analysis of case. *"The more general and undefined symptoms: loss of appetite, headache, debility, restless sleep, discomfort, and so forth, demand but little attention when of that vague and indefinite character, if they cannot be more accurately described, as symptoms of such a general nature are observed in almost every disease and from almost every drug".*

Kentian School: Dr. J. T. Kent analysed the sum total of case into General symptoms, Particular symptoms and the particular symptoms.

The General symptom is the one which is experienced by the patient as a whole while the particular symptom is the one that pertains to a part. *"The things that lie closest to man and big life, and his vital force, are the things that are strictly general, and as they become less intimately related to man they become less and less general, until they become particular"*.

Common symptoms are experienced by a large number of patients or provers and are of little value in remedy selection.

Dr. R. G. Miller in his booklet - On the Comparative Value of Symptoms categorically states that both generals and particulars may either be characteristic and particular" and vice versa.

Boenninghausian School: It was Dr. Boenninghausen who worked a great deal on the concept of Analysis of Symptoms. He gave clear directions as to how the physician should dismember the patient language into the complete symptom. He also contributed the "Doctrine of Analogy" to assist the physician in completing the symptoms. He advocated on giving priority to complete symptoms, which consists of: In

Location

Sensation

Modality

Concomitants

In Kent's method both symptoms & remedies are graded, while in Boenninghausen's method only remedies are graded and evaluated in therapeutic pocket book.

Dr. Boger's View: Dr. Boger held the view that the case should be scrutinized for the disease symptoms and the individual symptoms. It is these individual symptoms which hold a higher priority as they focus on the response of the vital force to the disease, thus characterizing the symptoms of the person. *"The final analysis of every case, therefore, resolves itself into the assembling of the individualistic symptoms into one group and collecting the disease manifestations into another, then finding the remedy which runs through both, while placing the greater emphasis on the former"*.

Dr. Sankaran's View: He classified symptoms into:

Pathognomonic Symptoms: Symptoms of the disease; helpful for diagnosing the case.

Non-Pathognomonic Symptoms: Symptoms of the patient which help us to select proper Homeopathic medicine.

The greater the value of a symptom in a diagnostic sense, the less its value in therapeutic sense.

Dr. Garth Boericke's View: Classification of symptoms into Basic (Common and Diagnostic) and Determinative (Characteristic and Guiding).

Basic or Absolute Symptoms or Pathognomonic Symptoms: Symptoms that appear in every proving and diseases and are important for diagnosis.

Determinative or Non-pathognomonic symptoms: These are strange, rare or peculiar symptoms of the patient, they are characteristic of an individual and are important for prescription.

It must be remembered that Dr. Boericke uses the term Basic Symptoms and

Determinative Symptoms to denote Common and Uncommon symptoms respectively; and Dr. Boenninghausen often uses the terms Primary Symptoms and Secondary Symptoms to express the same order meanings.

Dr. N. Ghatak's View: Dr. Ghatak divided the symptoms into Subjective and Objective symptoms. The subjective symptoms again classified in to personal (relating to the patient as a whole) and local symptoms (relating to localities).

Dr. G. I. Bidwell divides all symptoms from innermost to outermost, from mind to skin, from generals to particulars into two divisions

(a) Strange, rare, peculiar and uncommon symptoms; and

(b) The common symptoms

Though all may seem different yet the essence of all their teachings remains the same. Going through all the above views the student should not let himself get confused over which path to tread, for irrespective of the road he chooses he is bound to reach the Similimum safely provided he understands the underlying concept. To further simplify the intricacies of analysis I wholeheartedly support Dr. Roberts usage of words of famous detective character of Arthur Canon Doyle, Sherlock Holmes about acting as a scientific detective, *"That which is out of the common is usually a guide rather than a hindrance"*. Thus it is the uncommon which should be given more preference while analyzing the case. The final outcome of analysis should help the physician to extract the following information:

Causation: Ailments from, physical and emotional factors.

General modalities: Aggravations and ameliorations, relations to heat and cold.

Characteristic particulars (modalities, etc.)

Rare, peculiar and striking symptoms.

Concomitants.

Common symptoms with location, sensation and modalities.
Analysis and Evaluation

While Analysis is breaking up of the case recorded into viable constituents; Evaluation is the hierarchal enlisting of these units according to importance.

Analysis (*Breaking up of Whole into Parts*)
↓
Evaluation (*Enlisting of the parts according to importance*)
↓
Synthesis of Case (*Construction of Case*)
↓
Repertorisation
↓
Prescribing Similimum
↓
Cure

One thing to remember is that Analysis and Evaluation are always done based on certain school of philosophy. The process of analysis and evaluation is in fact, a sieving up of the case recorded in order to procure a complete ripe case which can be helpful in Repertorization.

E. DIFFICULTIES IN CHRONIC CASE TAKING

Case taking is essentially a social interaction between a physician and a patient under certain pre determined condition.

We have to face many difficulties because of the ignorance of the masses who are not accustomed to a detailed narration of their sufferings to enable us for a homoeopathic prescription. our task is made even more difficult by the easy methods adopted by the modern system of medicine.

Bringing the masses, who are accustomed to the easy methods and impressive instruments, to the simple but the surer method of cure is a difficult task. We must under stand that their can be no substitute for human brain and that no instrument can understand the human sufferings and only a human mind can realize the depth of the sufferings.

1. **The influence of modern system upon the people**

    A physician trained in modern methods of treatment does not trouble the patient much by way of asking questions for case taking. The patient who are accustomed to such procedure and influenced by these techniques, come to a homoeopath and expect him to follow the same procedure with out touching the patient much in the way of interrogation and prescribe medicine for his trouble, yet expecting to have better results.

2. **Changed symptom image**

    When all the possibilities of allopathic medicine including surgery fails, patient come to the homoeopath as their last resort. By the time he must have consumed large quantity of strong drugs continuously for a long time. The already consumed drug must have produced their own symptoms (drug proving) changing the symptoms image of original disease, thus making the homoeopathic physician incapable of making a radical prescription.

3. **Complex disease**

    Allopathic medicines are not prescribed according to the symptom similarity & are repeated quite often and unscientifically; when natural chronic disease are treated with these drugs, they produce their own symptoms (drug disease) and intimately mix with the already existing natural disease and cause complex disease which are very difficult to cure.

4. **When pathology progress the signs & symptoms decreases**

    Many disease such as cancer usually comes on later in life, when childhood matters have been forgotten, they don't remember the past history or family history. Pathological changes have already taken place. In proportion as the pathology progress ,the signs and symptoms decreases. In the absence of signs and symptoms/totality of symptoms the choice of the medicine is not possible and on pathology alone no prescription can be made.

5. **Modesty conceals the facts**

   There are certain conditions and sufferings which the patient may not like to disclose to the doctor due to modesty or shame. Due to modesty patient conceal the facts and give vague symptoms which make the correct prescription difficult. E.g. Habitual masturbation Leucorrhoea in females.

6. **Pretension modifies the symptoms**

   Certain patients exaggerate their symptoms, narrate more than they feels. Some patient narrate less than they feels. In certain grave diseases they don't complain about their sufferings. These are hinder the proper case taking.

7. **Patients accustomed to long sufferings**

   In chronic disease, the patient get accustomed to their long sufferings and may not feel the necessity of narrating the symptoms with which they have lived for long, which are important for the choice of medicine. They don't consider that these symptoms have anything to do with the prescription that has to be made for the present trouble.

8. **Symptoms appearing periodically are not narrated**

   Symptoms appearing periodically are important factors, which will help in the selection of medicine. The patient being ignorant of the importance of such symptoms occurring periodically along with the main symptoms may not narrate these while giving their case history. E.g. Rheumatism during winter Diarrhoea during rainy season.

9. **Alternating symptoms not narrated**

   Certain symptoms usually alternate with one another. They don't understand the important of such alternating symptoms; moreover they are not aware of such alternation, thus making the proper prescription impossible.

10. **The long sufferings considered incurable**

    The treatment for the new disease cannot be considered until a complete picture of the old symptoms is obtained. Due to gradual progress of the chronic disease, many symptoms are produced one after another, and with which the patient might have been living since long. During this course some serious diseases develops which are the result of the existing chronic disease. Patient ignoring of the old symptoms, thinking that they are incurable, seek treatment for the new disease. so the complete picture cannot be obtained.

11. **Un homoeopathic homoeopathic medicines**

    Some doctors usually prescribe complexes and tonics, eye drops and nasal drops to their patients. Each complexes/tonics contain 5-6 medicines. When they are administered, it will produce their own symptoms which will be more dangerous to the patient than natural disease. So that, it would not have been possible for the homoeopathic medicine to overpower the natural disease and cure it. (usually homoeopathic medicines are more powerful than natural chronic disease.

- Complexes and tonics are not prepared according to symptom similarity.
- They will produce their own symptoms (proving) and create a medicinal chronic diseases.
- This will mix up with the natural chronic disease and make a complex disease which will be incurable.

12. Self medication

If the patient get well by self medication, he does not come to a doctor. But if the symptoms remain, he come to the clinic. As a result of prolonged medication the symptom remain suppressed and cause a problem for the physician.

13. Mixed miasmatic disease

There are certain diseases which have a combination of psora, syphilis and sycosis in a complex; it is very difficult to penetrate in these cases.

14. One sided disease

These diseases present too few symptoms for a judicious prescription.

F. CONCEPT OF TOTALITY ACCORDING TO BOENNINGHAUSEN, BOGER AND KENT

A) BOENNINGHAUSEN'S CONCEPT OF TOTALITY:
In his concept totality of symptoms comprises following seven points.

- Quis Personality, the individuality
- Quid Disease, its nature and peculiarity
- Ubi Seat of the disease
- Quibus Auxilis Accompanying symptoms.
- Cur Cause of disease
- Quomodo Modification, agg. and amel.
- Quando Time

Philosophical background of Boenninghausen's repertory rests on the following.

1. Doctrine of Analogy
2. Doctrine of concomitance
3. Evaluation of remedies
4. Concordance

Doctrine of analogy: According to Boenninghausen one can make order out of chaos by combining the scattered symptoms by making use of analogy. To complete a symptom local maladies and sensations pertaining to one part should also be applied to other parts. Thus he raised local symptoms to a general level which could be used for the whole person this is called doctoring of grand generalization. He also evolved the concept that 'what is true to the part is also true to the whole person'. Boenninghausen's approach was that proving are not complete and can never be really complete.

He says that to make things comparatively more complete, so as to make the best of what can be found out; he wanted to complete the case by analogy as learned from actual experience and practice.

Doctrine of concomitant: The word concomitant means existing or occurring together; or attendant. They are the unreasonable attendants of the case. Boenninghausen identified in each case a group of symptoms which have no relation to the leading symptom from the standpoint of theoretical pathology, yet they have actual relationship with the case in that they exist in same person at the same time. Concomitant is the differentiating factor in any case. The foundation of the TPB lies in it.

Evaluation of remedies: Boenning Hausen was the first to grade the remedies, there are 5 gradings

CAPITALS marks FIRST GRADE	-	5
BOLD marks SECOND GRADE	-	4
ITALICS marks THIRD GRADE	-	3
ROMAN marks FOURTH GRADE	-	2
ROMAN (PARANTHESIS) FIFTH GRADE	-	1 mark

This gradation is based on frequency and intensity of the appearance of symptom in provers.

5 marks Symptom frequent, confirmed and verified

1 mark Symptom not verified, not confirmed

Concordance: In the earlier edition the headings is concordance of remedies, by changing Allen makes this more comprehensive. This chapter is divided into sections, each begin with a section devoted to a remedy in alphabetical order.

Each of these remedy section is subdivided into rubric Mind, Localities, Sensation, Glands, Bones, Skin, Sleep and Dreams, Blood; Circulation and Fever, Aggravation: Time and circumstances, Other remedies, Antidotes, Injurious. Other remedies mean general relationship of remedies. Other remedies also cover these symptoms which do not fit into the above said rubrics.

B. BOGER'S CONCEPT:

Dr. C. M. Boger in his book "Studies in the philosophy of healing" gives a scientific procedure for "choosing the remedy". According to him the characteristic symptom comprises following seven points

1. Change of personality and temperament: To be particularly noted when striking alterations occur.
2. Peculiarity of disease: e.g. Stepladder pattern in typhoid
3. Seat of the disease: Every drug acts more definitely upon certain parts of the organism; right, left, diagonally etc. e.g. Sepia cures stubborn abscess of fingers and toes.
4. Concomitance
5. Cause
6. Modalities
7. Time

A. Periodicity
B. Hour of the day when they are better or worse

Boger's work Boenninghausen's characteristics and repertory is based on the following fundamental concepts

1. Doctrine of complete symptom and concomitant
2. Doctrine of pathological general
3. Doctrine of causation and time
4. Clinical rubrics
5. Evaluation of remedies
6. Fever totality
7. Concordance

Doctrine of complete symptom and concomitant: A complete symptom is that which consists of location, sensation, modalities and concomitants. Boger borrowed this idea of complete symptom from Boenninghausen's method of erecting totality, but he improved it by relating sensation and modalities to specific parts, thereby he fairly and squarely met the criticism.

In the book, the complete symptoms are well arranged. Concomittnats are given greater importance by Boger in relation to parts.

Doctrine of pathological general: Pathological generals tell the state of the whole body and its changes in relation to the constitution. They help us to concentrate on more concrete changes to select the simillimum. The chapter in the book "sensations and complaints in general" is full of examples of pathological generals, which include discharges, structural alterations, constitutions, diathesis etc.

Doctrine of causation and time: From his point of view, causation and time factors are more definite and reliable in cases as well as in medicines. Each chapter in the book is followed by time aggravation. The section on aggravation also contains many causative factors. In the chapter 'choosing the remedy' he gives importance to the miasmatic cause, as well as exciting cause. In his hierarchy of evaluating symptoms he gave more importance to causation and general modalities.

Clinical rubrics: Boger mentioned several clinical rubrics in his repertory. These rubrics help the physician in cases of advanced pathology. These rubrics are useful to arrive at a group of medicines, which can further be narrowed down, with the help of modalities and concomitants to select finally the most similar remedy.

Evaluation of remedies: He introduced the grading of symptoms into five ranks by the use of different topography such as

- Capital 5
- Bold 4
- Italic 3
- Roman 2
- Roman in parenthesis (1), rarely used.

The gradation is based on the frequency of the appearance of symptoms in the provers. Thus five mark medicines are most important and one mark medicines least important.

Fever totality: This is the unique contribution of Boger. The arrangement is self explanatory. Each stage of fever is followed by time, aggravation, amelioration and concomitant. Thus they help to repertorize any simple as well as complicated cases of fever.

Concordance: By including this chapter Boger has made the philosophy clearer and practical. It deals with the relationship of 125 remedies.

C. KENTS PHILOSOPHY: Kent's repertory is based on philosophy of deductive logic. i.e. from generals to particulars. Generals are dealt within depth followed by particulars, and minute particulars. Under chapter mind mental generals are given. The physical generals are mostly listed under generalities, and a few in other chapters.

Kentian method: Dr. Kent has classified the symptoms into three main categories:

1. General
2. Particular
3. Common

1. **General symptoms:** All the symptoms that the patient predicate of himself or of which he uses the first person pronoun are general symptoms. e.g. I am weak, I am thirsty. As the general symptoms affect the patient as a whole they are of higher value.

General symptoms subdivided into two groups

A) Mental generals
   - Will and emotion
   - Understanding
   - Intellect

B) Physical generals:
   - Perversion of sexual sphere and effects of coition
   - Symptoms pertaining to appetite, food desires and aversions, thirst
   - Things affecting the entire body

- Weather
- Food
- Position
- Motion
- Symptoms of special senses

2. **Particular symptoms:** They refer to the symptoms related to a particular part of the body of the patient

   - First grade particular: Those that are rare and unusual e.g. inflammation without pain.
   - Second grade particular: Particular symptom with marked modalities.
   - Third grade particulars: Particular symptoms without modality.

3. **Common symptoms:** This symptom is common to a particular disease or is found in several patients as a common factor. They do not play much role in the selection of similimum unless they have peculiar modalities.

Kent's repertory contains 648 drugs and he has used three varieties of topography indicating the gradation of remedies.

Bold letter 3 marks First grade

Italics 2 marks Second Grade

Ordinary 1 mark Third grade.

Provers Reproved Verified

First grade symptoms ++++ ++++ ++++

(All provers) (Reproved) (Verified)

Second Grade ++ ++++ ++

(Few) (Reproved) (Occasionally verified)

Third grade + ---- +

(Occasionally) (Not seen) (Clinical symptom)

Though all the three are important, its relevance depends on the nature of the case.

G. PAEDIATRIC CASE TAKING

General instructions

- Physician should be soft, gentle, friendly & caring with genuine interest & love for children
- Be smiling & polite to children & never get angry with children even if they are at their worst
- Approach the child with a smiling face & treat him as a child & not as a patient & comfort him
- Never start examining the child as soon as he enters the clinic & try to build a rapport with the child before examination
- Should literally come down to the level of child both physically & mentally to elicit cooperation
- Clinic should be well lighted, quiet & decorated with toys & pictures to allay the anxiety of the child & can offer a soft toy to establish a rapport
- Questioning of the children should be avoided at the very beginning of the interview
- Ask the mother about the child's behavior, but observe the child constantly during the interview. Answers from the mother are less relevant than the observations you make while you are interviewing the mother
- But do not be tempted to interrupt a mother in full flow to try & ask what you think is a clever question; it will be like trying to impose our diagnosis on them

- Observation of each & every movement of the child should be noted properly & can spend maximum on it
- Intelligent neglect of the child & proper respect to the mother to gain the child's confidence is essential
- A careful observation during the interview often reveals stresses & concern which are otherwise not apparent
- We should confirm our observations by direct questioning or using leading questions & tricky questions which is essential & safe here
- For school going children asking them their name, name of school, age, hobbies, their best friend, name of their teacher etc makes them feel at ease
- Avoid staring at the child because they are often scared if you intently look into their eyes
- Anxiety of the parents should be allayed. Over anxious parents will ask many questions about the child. Proper explanation in context to the questions & relevant developmental milestones of a normal child along with its normal variations should be explained to allay the anxieties of parents
- Physicians should also observe the interactions between the child and parents. This reveals the amount of concern of the parents towards the child's health & interests. It also reveals the notion of do's & don'ts in the family of child

- To get the desired information, it is necessary to have privacy which is often overlooked in case of children as some adolescent children who are often rather resentful of their parents, will be happy to share their thoughts when alone
- Parents also will be interested to talk in private with doctor & often during such discussion that the real reason for consultation emerges
- Care should be taken not to ridicule, not to laugh at what the child says seriously, not to be always funny or amusing and not to tease unless the child is known well
- If the problem is related to the adjustment of the child or its behavior, parents & child should be given suggestions separately & or both together as deemed necessary
- In younger children the observation of parents & physician himself are utmost important
- In acutely ill child, information obtained rapidly and in brief may suffice to identify the primary problems of concerns
- The essence of art of examining children is that during the most of the examination the child should be contented

CASE TAKING IN DETAIL

There cannot be any standard or regulated patterns of history taking, as the questioning will change depending on the age group of the patient we are dealing with Physician should be aware about the normal physical, social, emotional & intellectual development.

Questions should be asked to understand the moral character, intellectual character, social & domestic relationships.

Data can be collected in an order of

1. **Chief complaints** – with causations like vaccinations, emotional turbulences, physical factors, medicines etc.

2. **History of present illness.**

3. **Associated complaints.**

4. **Past history** – of previous illnesses; their nature, severity, the age at which occurred, like infectious diseases, seizures, bowel disturbances, URTI, discharging ears, cough & history of accidents, physical injuries, burns or poisonous incidents and medical history.

5. **Prenatal history** i.e. mother's history during pregnancy - relevant in cases of congenital disorders, tumors, juvenile arthritis, juvenile diabetes.

   - Any illnesses she had? like rubella & any drug history
   - **Maternal stress**-emotional stress during pregnancy like anxieties, fear, tensions in relationship with husband & other family members, friends her reactions to that
   - Economic status of family
   - Attitude of not wanting a baby at all, or at that time

6. **Birth history**
   - How was the delivery-normal vaginal or forceps, breach, cesarean etc
   - Full term?
   - Birth weight
   - Enquiry about jaundice, breathing & feeding difficulties, fits etc

7. **History after birth**
- Was the mother unconscious after delivery
- How soon were the mother & child brought together after delivery

8. **Feeding history** - how often? how does suck the breast? fast or slow? any preference for side of breast?
- If bottle fed, which milk? Any diarrhoea, regurgitation, colic etc?
- When weaning started?
- If child asks for extra feeds & are not content with the quantity of mother's milk can consider as thirsty & others are thirstless

9. **Developmental history**
- Mile stones like smile, dentition, crawl, walk, talk etc
- Precocity
- assessment of intellect-intelligences of linguistic or verbal, logical or mathematical, bodily or kinesthetic, spatial or visual, musical or rhythmic etc.

10. **Immunization history**-when? how many times? which ?

11. **Family history**
- How old are the parents?
- How many children are there in family. their age, sex
- Any still births, miscarriages, or childhood deaths in family
- Any illnesses in siblings, parents or near relatives

12. **Social history**-Living conditions, economic status, mother's occupation

13. **Child as a person**-physical & mental characteristics, life situation.

14. **Physical Constitution**
- Distribution of fat
- Progress of emaciation
- Eating habits

a) **Physical generals** - Thermal state by checking temperature of abdomen, neck, perspiration, usage of covering during sleep
  - Appetite & thirst
  - Desires & aversions
  - Sleep-How does the child wake from sleep, sleep position,deep or light sleep

b) **Emotional level & expressions of reactions to stimuli**
  - Anger response-impulsive (extrapunitive & intrapunitive) or
  - Inhibited
  - Jealousy & its reactions-direct & indirect
  - Grief-expressive & non expressive
  - Fears- in babies (towards loud noises, dark rooms, animals, high places, strange persons, places, objects, being alone) in pres school children - (towards ghosts, monsters, darkness, sleeping alone inschool going children - school performance, results, reprimands)
  - Shyness, embarrassments, worry, anxiety with heir expression behaviour & temperamental patterns

c) **Sociability**
  - approach or withdrawal
  - adaptability

d) Activity

- Activity level-high or low
- Threshold of responsiveness (sensitivity) - to sound, taste, touch, temperature change
- Intensity of reaction-amount of energy a child uses to express emotions like High intensity denotes-laughing & crying loudly, is easily frustrated, screams so loud,
- Rhythmicity-regularity of biological functions like sleep, hunger & eliminations
- Distractibility - how much or how little extraneous stimulus is needed to interfere with an ongoing activity
- Attention span & persistence - how long a child can stay with any given activity

e) Destructabilty - destructive or non destructive

15. Thoughts on Miasms behind And can conclude the interview with general physical examinations with proper systemic & relevant local examinations.

H. CASE TAKING IN UNCONSCIOUS PATIENT

The unconscious patient can be a challenge in the pre hospital setting, where it is not always apparent or obvious what is causing the patient to be unconscious. There is always the potential that the patient is critically ill or injured and it is important to try to anticipate the potential cause of unconsciousness. Following is an overview of select causes of unconsciousness.

Acute Alcohol Intoxication

The amount of alcohol needed for a patient to become unconscious will vary with each case. Contributing factors include the volume of alcohol consumed, the rate of consumption, if the alcohol was ingested on an "empty stomach" and the individual's tolerance to alcohol. It may be reported that the patient was "binge" drinking, which is often associated with consuming an excessive amount of alcohol in a relatively short period of time.

Insulin

Patients who are taking insulin to manage their diabetes may have taken an excessive amount of insulin resulting in hypoglycemia. This can occur intentionally or accidentally. The patient may also be taking more than one medication that is intended to assist in maintaining a glucose level within a certain range. If the medications are administered incorrectly or out of normal sequence with a schedule, it is possible for the patient's blood glucose level to drop very quickly to an acutely low or abnormally low level and the patient may lose consciousness. Left uncorrected, hypoglycemia, or low blood sugar, can have serious consequences for the patient.

Drug Overdose

An individual may become unconscious following excessive consumption of a prescribed or over-the-counter medication or as the result of overdosing on a "street" drug, such as heroin. The list of possible scenarios that might be involved in a drug overdose situation is extensive. In some cases it may be unclear as to what drug/medication was taken, when it was taken, or how much was ingested. As an EMS provider, you should recall that routes of ingestion and drug forms vary. Common routes of ingestion include oral, nasal, intravenous and smoke inhalation. Drug forms can include pill, powder, fluid and drugs combined with other substances like a paste or other solutions. Depending on the situation, it might not be possible to determine which drugs are involved until the patient can be evaluated in an emergency department.

Trauma

In the pre hospital setting, in either blunt or penetrating trauma cases, it is not always possible to determine the specific injury or injuries involved. It is, however, essential that you are able to quickly recognize that the patient has a serious injury that may be causing unconsciousness. Examples include hypovolemia from internal and external hemorrhage, organ rupture, injury to the central nervous system (brain and spinal cord) and massive chest injuries. Management of the unconscious trauma patient may be limited in the pre hospital setting, as surgical intervention may be necessary. The unconscious trauma patient should always be considered a candidate for a trauma center until proven otherwise.

Psychiatric Disorders

While some causes of unconsciousness, such as a gunshot wound to the head, may be obvious, psychiatric causes or emergencies may be subtle. In suspected or confirmed cases of psychiatric disorders combined with unconsciousness, you will need to carefully and thoroughly assess the patient. If witnesses or bystanders are available, try to elicit a thorough history of events and ask specific interview questions. This may prove to be invaluable in assisting with a treatment plan. Examples of interview questions, which can be applied in almost any unconscious patient encounter, include: Has the patient been unconscious before? What was the cause? Could substance abuse or trauma be involved? Does the patient have any additional underlying medical conditions? What was the patient doing prior to becoming unconscious?

Neurological

An acute stroke can result in unconsciousness for any patient. Signs and symptoms will vary based on factors like the nature and location of the stroke. As with any unconscious patient, the patient's underlying health will also be a factor. Stroke can be caused by ischemic cerebral events as well as hemorrhagic events. In the pre hospital setting it is not possible to determine the type or location of a stroke when the patient is unconscious.

Infection

An infection can result in unconsciousness and may present subtly. EMS may be called to assess an individual who appears lethargic, excessively tired or perhaps "not normal". In these situations, a thorough medical history and patient assessment are important. Subtle findings like febrile skin, tachycardia and tachypnea may be present. The presence of additional injuries, such as open infected wounds, should also be noted. The patient with a systemic infection may require intensive care that exceeds the scope of pre hospital care.

Summary

Information about patient can be collected from following sources while taking a case:-

a) The Physical Examination.

b) Investigations.

c) Interrogation of friends and relatives.

When a patient is unconscious, a thorough assessment will be invaluable when attempting to identify a possible cause. A detailed assessment will also assist you in developing a potential treatment plan. Treatment of the unconscious patient will vary with each situation. Providers should always focus on supporting the patient's airway, breathing and circulation, and supplemental oxygen should be administered.. In cases where trauma is suspected or confirmed, cervical spine precautions should be taken. Hospital destination will be influenced by a variety of factors, including if the incident is due to a medical or traumatic event.

I. THE ANAMNESIS AND CATAMNESIS

ANAMNESIS

Origin:

It is a Greek word which means "recalling". Anamnesis is etymologically a derivative form of Mnemosyne who was the Greek Goddess of memory.

Definition:

Anamnesis as a tool of case perceiving is used in homoeopathy in a broader sense than just medical history as it involves recalling of all the past happenings especially the painful and traumatic events.

INTRODUCTION

Anamnesis may be defined as medical or psychiatric history obtained from the patient, especially in the patient's own words, based on the recollections of events preceding his or her own illness.

In other words, it is an exposition of one's sickness from the recall to memory of the past occurrences and events.

In homoeopathic parlance, anamnesis is also termed as longitudinal case study. It is a mode of perceiving the evolution of presenting complaints and appreciating the effect of past in the development of present illness. Master Hahnemann underscored the importance of this concept of anamnesis or longitudinal case study in §5 of his 'Organon of Medicine' wherein he stated that, "Useful to the physician in assisting him to cure are the particulars of the most probable exciting cause of the acute disease, as also the most significant points in the whole history of the chronic disease, to enable him to discover its fundamental cause", Hahnemann further highlighted the significance of evolutionary case study in his

article 'Medicine of Experience' where in he emphasized that, "The internal essential nature of every malady, of every individual case of disease, as far as it is necessary for us to know it, for the purpose of curing it, expresses itself by the symptoms, as they present themselves to the investigation of the true observer in their whole extent, connection and succession".

Catamnesis - The study of follow-up of case is called catamnesis. In homoeopathy a detailed study of anamnesis and catamnesis is required.

Significance:

1) It helps to understand the case and help in correct prescribing.

2) It is required in chronic cases which begin after an acute attack.

3) To manage Periodic diseases.

4) It helps to understand familial disposition to the recurrence of certain form of disease at a certain period.

5) To see the progress of Alternating diseases.

SECTION II

A. INTRODUCTION TO REPERTORY

REPERTORY

A repertory is a place where information is stored or categorized so that it can be retrieved more easily. It is an index of symptoms, with a listing of all of the remedies known to be associated with each particular symptom. This information can be stored in a book format, on software, compact disc, or through a collection of cards (card repertories). The word "repertory" comes from the Latin word *repertus,* which means "to find".

The word 'repertory' means a store house, a store or collection especially of facts or information. The word originated from the Latin word REPERTORIUM or (REPERTIRE) which means "an inventory, a table or a compendium where the information is so arranged that it is easy to find. But the word "REPERTIRE" in French means a company store house.

"The meaning of repertory given in certain book as store house or inventory is a misnomer", Benedict D'Castro. According to him the word originates from the latin word REPERTORIUM. Repertorium is again derived from the Latin word REPERTUS, means reproduction. Repertory is an index of symptoms of materia medica, the record of scientific proving which is reproduced and artistically arranged in a practical form, indicating the relative gradation of medicines to facilitate the quick selection of the indicated medicines.

"Repertory is an index to the homoeopathic materia medica, which is full of informations collected from toxicology, drug proving, and clinical experience", says Dr. Tiwari. Repertory bridges the gap between materia medica on one hand and the disease on the other. Thus the study of repertory helps us to understand the patient and the materia medica. Materia medica and repertory are complement to each other.

PURPOSE OF THE REPERTORY

The purpose of the repertory is to help you find the right remedy for a given case. It is a tool. The repertory helps to individualize a case to find the right remedy for the right person. It also assists the practitioner find small and rarely used remedies and to link unusual symptoms with the appropriate remedy. There are some cases where using the repertory is crucial to finding the right remedy and other cases where it is much less useful.

HISTORY OF REPERTORIES

Initially in homeopathy there were no repertories. Hahnemann had only proven a few remedies, and it was possible to remember the symptoms that were associated with each of the known remedies. As further provings were undertaken and homeopathic knowledge increased, it was no longer possible to remember all the symptoms associated with each particular remedy. Repertories became increasingly necessary.

The first repertory was created by Hahnemann in 1805 and was handwritten. It was difficult to use, reflecting more an alphabetical index to the provings, and Hahnemann was never entirely happy with it. The next repertory to come out was written by Clemens Maria Boenninghausen in 1832. It was called *Repertory of Anti-psorics* and focused on the importance of modalities (something that makes a particular condition better or worse). Georg Jahr also wrote a repertory in 1835 called the *Symptomen-Codex*; it also was handwritten. This repertory was only based on proving symptoms. Hempel translated Jahr's repertory into English and added to it, creating a much more substantial repertory in 1848. The first French repertory was written by Lafitte in 1844 (*Symptomatologie homoeopathique, ou tableau synoptique de toute la matiere medicale pure.* Vol. I, Paris). Lippe was one of the first homeopaths to add more mental and emotional symptoms to the repertory. His repertory was expanded by Lee, who abandoned the effort when he went blind. Much of Kent's *Repertory* is based on the work of Lee and Lippe. Card repertories were popular in India. There have been more than 300 repertories created. Many are complete repertories, while others focus on only a specific area. These repertories are of varying quality and usefulness.

MODERN REPERTORIES

In more recent years efforts have been made to create repertories that are easier to use, which update the archaic language of many of the older repertories. Two of the most important of these are the *Complete Repertory* by Roger Van Zandvoort and the *Synthetic Repertory* by H. Barthel and W. Klunker. Both of these repertories are more expensive, but extensively researched, painstakingly constructed, and well designed. Robin Murphy's *The Homeopathic Medical Repertory* is also popular, although considerably shorter. Many of the newer repertories combine older repertories and add symptoms gained from more recent provings. Electronic versions of repertories are becoming increasingly common. Still, Kent's *Repertory of the Homeopathic Materia Medica* remains the most common repertory used in the world today. This workbook uses Kent's *Repertory* as its main reference.

INFORMATION ADDED TO THE REPERTORIES

The repertories are incomplete. There is always more information that needs to be added. The repertories are primarily based on symptoms obtained from provings. Another method in which remedies and symptoms are added to the repertory is through cured cases. When homeopaths consistently see a symptom cured by a particular remedy, this may be added to the repertory. You may also see information in the repertory that is based on accidental poisonings. These symptoms are then recorded into the repertory. One of the advantages of electronic homeopathic repertories is that this information can be updated much more quickly and regularly.

GRADING OF SYMPTOMS

When a proving is completed, the symptoms of that particular remedy are added to the repertory on a graded basis. Symptoms that are very strong, clear, and common are added as threes (3) (usually designated by dark and bold type); symptoms less common and only moderately clear and strong are added as twos (2) (usually designated by italics or plain type with underlining); symptoms that are infrequent and weaker in intensity are added as ones (1) (usually designated by plain type).

For example, on p. 37 of Kent's *Repertory*, you will find the heading of "Disgust". Puls (*Pulsatilla*) and Sulph (*Sulphur*) are listed in bold type for this particular symptom (3). Merc (*Mercurius vivus*) is the only remedy listed in italics (2) and Ars (*Arsenicum album*), Cimx (*Cimex*), Coloc (*Colocynthis*), Mez (*Mezereum*) and Phos (*Phosphorous*) are listed in plain type (1).

B. THE EVOLUTION OF REPERTORIES

History & Evolution of Repertory

As old as history of homoeopathy it has started with an appendix in 1805. Today it had grown to a system.

GROWTH _ 3 STAGES

1. Formative years : From Hahnemann to Kent
2. Middle age : Kentian era
3. Recent repertories : Software based

EARLIER REPERTORIES

Many where kept in Hale's museum in Robert Bosch Hospital, Stuttagret, West Germany.

1805. Appendix to Fragmenta de Viribus Medica Mentarum Positivus. (second part Dr. Hahnemann) Drug name _ Symptoms with modalities only ; no rubrics.

1814. Short repertory in latin by Dr. Hahnemann.

1828. Repertory in German by Hart laub & Trink.

1828. Repertory in 2 Vol. by Hahnemann (Each with 1000 pages) In German _ Manuscript form Considerd as forerunner of subsequent repertories.

1829. Repertory of Ernst Ferdinand Ruckert.

Around 1829_30. WEber's repertory with preface by Hahnemann (529 pages), Systemic work of Antipsoric remedies (Syste matische Darstellung Antipsoriche Arznemittal) Around 1829. Rep by Gustar W Gross

1829. Frederick Jacob Rummel - Incomplete repertory.

1832. Boenninghausen's Repertory of Anti psoric with a preface by Hahnemann.

1833. Glazor. First alphabetical pocket repertory (165 pages)

1833. Weber Peschier _ Repertory of purely pathogenitic effects with a preface by Hahnemann.

1835. Boenninghausen's Rep. of medicines which are not antipsorics.

1835. Repertory in 2 vol. by Dr.Jahr (1052+1254 pages)

1835. Rep. of Glands, Bones,Mucus Membrane, Ducts & Skin disease by Dr. Jhar (200 pages)

1836. Boennighausen _ Ver wand Schaften repertorium.

1837. Ruoff _236 pages

1843. Laffite French rep. of Syptamatology (975 pages)

1845. Ruoff _ A repertory of Nosology.

1845. Boenninghause's Therapeutic Pocket Book.

1847. Hemple's Boenninghausen's repertory (500 pages)

1848. Clofarmuller (940 pages)

1849. Mure. R (367 pages)

1851. Bryant. An alphabetical repertory (352 pages)

1853. Possart.A rep. of chtics. Homoeopathic remedies (700 pages)

1854. A. Lippe. A repertory of comparative materia medica.

1859. Cipher. Repertory by English Homoeopaths.

1873. Berridge.Repertory of Eye.

1874. Homoeolexicon by Granier of Nimes.

1879. C. Lippe. Rep. of more Chtics. symptoms of MM.

1880. T. F. allen's syptom register (Allentown register)

1881. Herring's Analytical repertory.

1890. Gentry. The Rep. of Concordances in 6 vol. (5500 pages)

1896. Knerr's repertory of Herring's Guiding symptoms.

1897. Kent's repertory. 1st edition (1349 pages)

ERA OF REGIONAL REPERTORIES (1880 - 1900)

Many of them were clinical repertories. Important among are...

1880. Repertory of Fever by H. C. Allen.

Sensation as if by H. A. Robert.

Repertory of Modalities by

Worcester.

Repertory of Intermittent Fever by W. A. Allen.

Repertory of Haemorroids by Guernesy.

1894. Rheumatism by Porlunins.

1899. Repertory of Urinary organs by Morgan.

1900. Repertory of Back by Wilsy.

1906. Repertory of uterine therapeutics by Minton.

Repertory of Diarrhoea by Bell.

1906. Rep. part of Raue's special pathology.

Repertory by Boerick.

Clark's clinical repertory.

Repertory of Mastitis by W. J. Gurnesy.

BOGER'S CONTRIBUTION TO REPERTORY

1900. Transalation of repertory of Antipsorics.

1905. Boger Boenn. Chrtics. Repertory

1906. Moon phases & Times of remedies.

1928. Symptamatology of Homoeopathic MM & Repertory.

1933. Genaral analysis & Card repertory.

CARD REPERTORY

1829. Guernesy's Boenninghause's slips (1st card repertory)

Based on Therapeutic Pocket Book.

_ Allen's Boenninghausen's slips by H. C. Allen.

1912. M. L. Tyler. Punched card repertory based on Kent.

1913. Dr. Welsch & Houstom. Loose punch card based on Kent.

1922. Dr. Field's card repertory (Best card repertory 6800 cards)

1928. Boger's card repertory.

1951. Dr. Marcoz jemenes. 1st to introduce gradation (600 cards)

1957. Dr. Sankaran's card repertory based on Boger.

1959 . Dr. Jugal Kishores card repertory.

INDIA'S CONTRIBUTION :

Phenominal...Bad _ Mutilated by men like K. C. Mittal who stole Kent's 7th edition from Pierrie Schmidt.

1978. Kent's 7th edition 2 vol.

1980. Kent's final general repertory by Dr. Diwan Harischand & P. Schmidt.

Dr. R. P. PATEL

1st to give index to Kent's repertory (as big as Kent's repertory)

Introduced computer from Australia to India (1967-68)

Introduced corrected version of Kent's repertory.

Standardized abbreviations of Drugs.

Introduced Auto visual repertory.

ERA OF COMPUTER REPERTORIES:

Homeopathic Software are the entire set of programs, procedures, and routines associated with the operation of a computer system to analyze patients' cases in clinics. Following is the list of available Homeopathic softwares worldwide:

1. KHA's Mac Repertory and ReferenceWorks
2. **RADAR** / RadarOpus
3. **HOMPATH**
4. Complete Dynamics / Complete Repertory
5. **CARA** / ISIS
6. Diagnozit
7. Cough & Cold Prescriber by Dr. Rajesh Shah
8. Homeopathy Pro
9. Homeopathic Remedy Finder
10. Akiva
11. Earth's Remedy
12. Repertorium Homeopathicum digital II
13. Boger Comparative Software
14. AtamA Homeopathic Software
15. BOENNREP repertory
16. The "Duprat" expert system
17. Homeopathy Software by Zentrum Publishing
18. Stimulare

C. ANALYSIS & EVALUATION OF SYMPTOMS FOR REPERTORIZATION

Analysis of the Case:

It is nothing but the case study about its content for the appropriate treatment by

1. Master Hahnemann's classification of disease.
2. Master Hahnemann's classification of miasms

Classification of disease i.e. Indisposition / dynamic / Surgical / one sided / local diseases help in fitting of case for homoeopathy or not. Acute / Chronic / Acute excerbation of chronic diseases diagnosis help in selection of the specific symptoms for totality. After the Analysis of the case,

Analysis of the symptoms is to be done to the case fitting for Homoeopathy.

Defination of Analysis of Symptoms: "It is the breakdown of the all symptoms of the case into qualified/characteristic and unqualified/common symptoms and selection of only qualified/characteristic symptoms into various groups, from the case". As a result, each symptom can be evaluated for rearranging the only characteristic symptoms to erect the totality/ the conceptualization of image of the patient. Dr. J. N. Kanjilal and Dr. R. P. Patel have shown the way to break the case into:

1. **Dr. J. N. Kanjilal** in his book "Repertorization" categorize the symptoms as:

General		Particulars of Local	
Uncommon	**Common**	**Uncommon**	**Common**
Peculiar,	(Basic, Primary)	Peculiar,	(Basic, Primary)
Charecteristic,	1st Grade	Characteristic,	1st Grade
Individualising,	2nd Grade	Individualising,	2nd Grade
(Determinative,	3rd Grade	(Determinative,	3rd Grade
Secondary)		Secondary)	
1st Grade		1st Grade	
2nd Grade		2nd Grade	
3rd Grade		3rd Grade	

Dr. R. P. Patel in his book "The Art of Case Taking and Practical Repertorisation" classifies the symptoms as:

1. General
   i) Mental Generals
      a) **Rare, Uncommon, Peculiar, Striking (RUPS),**
      b) Common

   ii) Physical Generals:
      a) **Rare, Uncommon, Peculiar, Striking (RUPS),**
      b) Common

2. Particular
   i) **Rare, Uncommon, Peculiar, Striking (RUPS)**
   ii) Common

3. Common
   i) **Rare, Uncommon, Peculiar, Striking ((RUPS)**
   ii) Common to disease.

Dr. M. L. Dhawale in his book "Principles & Practice of Homoeopathy" breaks the symptoms as:

i)   Cause
ii) Aggravations
iii) Ameliorations
iv) Unexpected deviations, Cravings and Aversions and finally
v)   Characteristic particulars (Location, Sensation, Modalities & Concomitants)

After studying the all these three stalwarts view, it is my recommendation to classify all general symptoms into Qualified (defined) and Unqualified (undefined) and Particulars as Characteristic and Common and then selection of all qualified (Defined) Generals and Characteristic particulars categorization can be done as follows by renovation:

1. Cause (Mental & Physical)
2. Aggravations (Psycho-social & Physical)
3. Ameliorations (Psycho-social & Physical)
4. Unexpected deviations(Mental, Physical & Pathological Generals by PQRS), Pathological Generals, Cravings and Aversions (Mentally desired for crowd or solitude, work or rest & Physical for work or rest, thermals, foods which should be included by intensity) and finally
5. Characteristic particulars (Location, Sensation, Pathology, Discharges, Modalities & Concomitants).

Mental General concomitant if any.

These are nothing but the Qualified Mentals.

Physical General

Menstruation & Other Discharges	Peculiarity Modality:	Example: Vicarious menstruation
		Example: Agg. during menses
		Example: Amel. during mense
	Intensity:	Example: No mense or Menstruating twice in month
		Example: Heavy bleeding / less bleeding
Sex regarding	Peculiarity	Example: Increased sex desire with impotency
	Modalities	Example: Aggravation before, during, after coition. Amelioration after coition
		Intensity Example: Nymphomania, Sex desire[+++]
Aversions	Peculiarity, Modality, Intensity	
Desires	Peculiarity, Modalities, Intensity	
Thermals	Peculiarity, Modalities, Intensity	

Physical general concomitant if any.

- These are nothing but the defined Physical generals.
- Pathological generals if any, with peculiarity, modality and intensity.
- Characteristic Particular
- Peculiarity in location: One cheek red, other pale, Head more hot
- Peculiarities in Modalities: Pain of hand aggravated by slight touch but ameliorated by pressure.
- Differential modalities
- Peculiarity in sensation: Non-exhausting diarrhea
- Modalities: Agg. by heat or cold, foods, climate, specific time.
- Amel.by heat or cold, foods, climate, specific time.
- Intensity: of pain^{+++}, radiation, wandering etc.

Particular concomitant if any.

- **Pathology:** Peculiarity: Example: Painless ulcer
- Modalities: Example: Relation to heat & cold, foods.
- Intensity: Rapidly growing tumor or ulcer etc.

Discharges: Colour, Odour, Consistency, Mode of Onset.

- Peculiarity: Examples: Changeable colour, absent of required colour
- Modalities: Examples:Aggravation or Amelioration by it.
- Intensity: Examples: Amount^{+++}, Frequent^{+++} or No or less.

Utility of Analysis of symptoms

To avoid the unnecessary data in Erecting Totality, Eliciting Repertorial Syndrome, Selection of Symptoms for PDF, we need the analysis of symptoms.

Master Hahnemann's instructions help us for Analysis of symptoms. While case taking Master Hahnemann in aphorism 84 instruct us not to intrupt in middle while the patient is telling his story which may break the flow of thought and if broken the second time the flow of thought may come in different manner. Again in aphorism 85 he tells to give a demarcation line at the end of every symptom and some space before the demarcation line so that the unrevealed problems can be completed asking the questions. So the case is having full important and unimportant symptoms for homoeopathic prescription out of which we have to choose only the characteristic symptoms as per the aphorism 5 and 153. In aphorism 5, master tells us to consider the exciting causes in acute diseases and fundamental causes in chronic diseases which are nothing but the chronic miasms. In chronic cases, Mater instructs us to consider the physical constitution, moral and intellectual character, social and domestic relations, occupation, habits etc. but simultaneously warn us to be alert in taking the characteristic symptoms in mental, physical and behavioural level in the aphorism 153 of 6th edition of Organon while praising Boenninghausen is as follows:

"The more general & undefined symptoms; loss of appetite, headache, debility, restless sleep, discomfort, and so forth, demand but little attention when of that vague & indefinite character, if they can't be more accurately described, as symptoms of such a general nature are observed in almost every disease & from almost every drug".

So in analysis of symptoms we first break down the case to its Undefined Generals and Qualified Generals, Common Particulars and Characteristic particulars, then classify the Qualified generals to the category of 1st , 2nd grade and 3rd grade mental generals and physical generals to 1st, 2nd grade and 3rd grade physical generals, and lastly particulars to 1st , 2nd and 3rd grade particulars. The 1st grade mental generals are the qualified mental symptoms of Will and Emotion, the 2nd grade mental generals are the qualified mental symptoms of Intellect and Understanding, the third grade mental symptoms are the qualified mental symptoms of Memory. The mental symptoms are qualified by 1. Peculiarity, 2. Modality, 3. Intensity. Similarly 1st grade physical generals are the qualified physical symptoms of menstruation and sexual sphere, the second grade physical generals are the qualified physical symptoms of reaction to environment e.g., thermals, foods. The third grade physical generals are desires and aversions in relation to food and climate, and any abnormal functioning in relation to urination, bowel habit, thirst, and appetite as per the Dr. Bidwell.

The analysis of particular symptoms should be considered after breaking the particular symptoms into Causation, Pathology with or without discharges, Sensation, Location, Modalities and concomitants as per the instruction of Boenninghausen. The 1st grade particulars are the pathology with or without discharges / sensation with peculiarity, the 2nd grade particulars are the pathology with or without discharges/sensation with causations or modalities and the 3rd grade particulars are the pathology with or without discharges/ sensation with intensity.

Evaluation of symptoms

View of the different stalwarts for defining evaluation of symptoms:

1. **Dr. R.P.Patel:** The principles of grading or ranking of different kinds of symptoms in order of priority which are to be matched with the drug symptoms in order to cover the characteristic totality in a natural disease condition with that of the drug disease.

2. **Dr. J.N. Kanjilal:** Assessing the relative values of each item of vast collected materials.

3. **Dr. M.L. Dhawale:** "The classification that he accepts will indicate this evaluation". The example of the classification is given in analysis of symptoms.

Thus it is the grading by priority of the characteristic symptoms with comparison to other characteristic symptoms as per the school of philosophy.

Boenninghausen's Evaluation as per Dr. Robert

- Concomitant if any is highest as it decides the totality (Fever, Menstruation).

- A complete symptom is the grand symptom.

- Grand generalization is done.

- No differentiation is made among general concomitant to particular & general complete symptoms to particular complete symptoms.

PDF: Mental symptoms are kept for differentiation.

- Among the components of symptom

- Causation/Modality is prime importance.
- The intensified specific sensations.
- The specific Location values last.

Boenninghausen's Evaluation as per Dr. M. L. Dhawle

1. Causative Modalities: Emotional, Intellectual, Physical.
2. General Aggravations : Emotional, Intellectual, Physical.
3. General Ameliorations : Emotional, Intellectual, Physical.
4. Physical Generals : Sensations and Complaints.
5. Concomitants.
6. Mentals: For reference and differentiation.

Evaluation of qualified symptoms as per Kentian School

1. **Qualified Mentals** by Peculiarity, Modality and Intensity:

Will	1st grade mental
Understaning	2nd grade mental
Memory	3rd grade mental

2. **Defined Physical General** by Peculiarity, Modality and Intensity:

Menstruation & Other Discharges	1st grade physical general
Sex regarding	1st grade physical general
Gen. Agg.	2nd grade physical general
Aversions	3rd grade physical general
Desires	3rd grade physical general

3. **Limited Generalisation of Particulars**

   PDF: Charecteristic Particular

PQRS	1st grade particulars
Modalities	2nd grade particulars
Highly Intensified sensation	3rd grade particulars

Evolution of Kent's Concept of Totality:

Dr. Phelan's irrelevant interrogation unrelated to disease for his wife's Insomnia, irritated & astonished Dr. Kent.

i) How the physical and mental aspect of the person unrelated to the disease help in cure in the treatment of Homoeopathy ?

ii) He developed an earnest desire to learn truth behind those so irrelevancy used in Homoeopathy.

iii) He learned Homoeopathy, Dr. Hahnemann's portrait of disease formulation by Mental & Physical characteristic symptoms (δ – 5,7 & 153), the miasm portrait and Swedenberg's hierarchy of decedent of Aura in the hierarchy of Soul → Mind → Body.

iv) Then he gave his own theory of disease formation as follows:

Mental Itch →Vital force → Mind → Body.

Derrangement of Vital Force by pollution of Mind.

Behaviour is altered (Mind of Latent Psora)

Physical reaction to environment is altered. Then only Full pledged Latent Psora causes the disease later to the that organ which is weak.

The Evolution of Boger's Concept

1. Dr. Cyrus Maxwell Boger was a allopath by profession and was German in origin, and had been settled in America.

2. He learned Homoeopathy at the juncture when Boenninghausen school was criticised by Kentian school for his doctrine of grand generalisation & generalisation of concomitants and Kent was also criticised by Overgeneralisation mind, & over particularisation of extrimities. Both the schools had been claiming their accuracy through clinical case studies through the publications in journals, magazines etc.

3. In stead of supporting the one school, he studied the original German literature of Boenninghausen and also literature of Kent.

4. Boger took best from both the schools and eliminated the criticised concept. Thus Kentian Concept fitted to Bonninghausen's Format

5. He illustrated it in the hierarchy form in FOREWARD of Synoptic Key and in Studies in the Philosophy of Healing.

6. Unlike the Boenninghausen, he gave qualified mental symptoms high value and kept for repertorisation.

7. Like the Boenninghausen, he followed his format of giving high values to Causation and Modality of Mental symptoms than Mental state.

8. Similarly General Modality was given high value than Gen.sensation.

9. Boenninghausen's Grand Generalisation was eliminated & Kent's Limited Generalisation was used in repertorisation.

10. Generalisation of concomitant was also rejected.

11. The Concept of Pathological General was introduced by reasoning out the structural deviation at tissue level. One step ahead than the Miasm.

Boger's School of Evaluation (The era of Modernisation in Repertorisation by bridging Kent and Boenninghausen schools: Kentian Concept in Boenninghausen's format).

1. **Causations and Modalities:**
   - Pathological Generals
   - Mental Causation / Modalities
   - Physical Causation / Modalities

2. **Generals:**

   Qualified Mental state by Concomitant, Peculiarity, and Intensity.

   Defined Physical generals by Concomitant, Peculiarity, and Intensity.

   Sexual impulse
   - Menstruation and
   - Other discharges with concomitants if any
   - Aversion
   - Desires
   - Thermals, Fever with concomitants if any.
   - Thirst
   - Appetite

3. **Limited generalization of particulars can be done to upgrade into Generals.**

4. **Characteristic Particulars:**
   - Particular concomitant
   - PQRS symptoms
   - Modalities
   - Intensifies sensation

Differentiation: Any rubric can be differentiating factor as per high value. The General concomitant if any can decide the similimum remedy from totality in chronic case management and particular concomitant if any can decide the similimum remedy from sector totality in acute case management.

Conclusion: Proper Evaluation of symptoms is necessary for the erecting totality as per the philosophy of Repertory the case is adapted to. Even with the same set of symptoms, totality/conceptual image by Boennighausen Philosophy, Kentian Philosophy and Boger's Philosophy differ. Thus in case of the cross – repertorisation, without changing the totality and again the erection of totality as per the philosophy of that repertory is required through the evaluation for comparative study

D. STEPS TO REPERTORIZATION

Repertorisation is not only a mechanical process of counting rubrics and totaling marks obtained by a medicine, it also includes the logical steps to reach the repertory proper and finally differentiating the remedies with the help of Materia Medica. Repertory follows the logic of Induction & Deduction. The steps to repertorisation start from case taking and end by finding out simillimum. They are:

1) **Case taking.**

2) **Recording and interpretation.**

3) **Defining the problem.**

4) **Classifications and evaluation of symptoms.**

5) **Erecting totality.**

6) **Selection of repertory and repertorisation proper.**

7) **Repertorial result.**

8) **Analysis and prescription.**

CASE TAKING

Dr. Kent once mentioned to his followers, 'There are lot of symptom, but there is no case'. What is the case then ? A case comprises of symptoms which, gives the totality of a person's suffering. The totality of symptoms, forms a case for the physician. In every event there exists a totality provided an expert can perceive it; likewise, in every alteration of state of health a totality exists which can be perceived by a physician.

Case taking is the first step, and the outcome of treatment entirely depends upon the success of this first step. Any mistake committed here would certainly interfere in the selection of drugs and planning of the treatment.

A physician should be clear about his job in the beginning itself and must possess a clear understanding about the case. For Homoeopathic physician, expressions at all levels, mental, physical, general and particular, are required to individualize the person as well as to diagnose the condition. If this is clear in the beginning, case taking will be on the right lines. It is a unique art of getting into conversation, of serving and collecting data from patient as well as from the bystanders to define the patient as a person and disease. The purpose is to understand both the person and the disease. This particular method and approach is different from other systems of medicine.

There has been much discussion on case taking by many stalwarts and this subject has been dealt-with at length but still many make mistakes while applying this art in practice. This being an art, the individual skill plays an important role in applying the rules of case taking. It is difficult to apply a uniform standard in all the cases and in respect of all physicians. In case taking, physician applies his ability and skills of communication keeping in view his objective. As case taking is individualized in approach, there are several suggestions offered and numerous models of case taking forms are available to the practitioners. Some are in the form of questionnaires, some in the form of multiple choice questions, and so on. Dr Dhawale has devised a Standardized Case Record which has a fixed form, structure and function. It can be most useful to the profession if used properly.

Dr Hahnemann has described the necessary guidelines which should be taken into consideration while taking a case, in aphorisms 83-104 of Organon of Medicine. Throughout the process of case taking, the patient should be cooperative. He should be assured of the confidentiality of data. If patient narrates well and fully, the task becomes easier for the physician. Apart from the collection of data, case taking has got its own therapeutic value in certain type of cases, if not all. Personal experience in certain cases has convinced the author about the therapeutic value of it. Many patients ventilate certain experiences unexpressed for years which keep on disturbing them and giving rise to very many physical and mental symptoms. Very often after the case taking, the patient says, "Doctor, I feel much relieved after talking to you", and then a simillimum completes its job. It should be a free exchange between the patient and the physician. Both verbal and non-verbal communication of the physician can either encourage or discourage the patient in opening up various events and their effects on him. It is a very delicate, yet dynamic situation, where the physician should remain attentive so that disclosures are properly received. Physician should be aware of is own problems of communication to gain more from this highly dynamic process. In some cases, even if one thread is missed, arriving at the totality would become difficult. Nothing else should keep the physician occupied other than the case taking. To understand the feelings properly, a physician should be expert in role playing. He should acknowledge the feelings of the patient, but empathy should replace sympathy while dealing with sensitive cases. At the end of the interview with the patient, physician should have a clear definition of the problem. This is not always easy to achieve. If physician remains in confusion at the level of case taking, further steps in repertorisation would become intractable. A shaky foundation would certainly mar even the best of the superstructure.

RECORDING AND INTERPRETATION:

Need of a case record has been emphasized by all the stalwarts for various essential purposes. Every case can be a piece of learning. Therefore, it is imperative to have it recorded properly. Since it is almost impossible to keep all the data intact without any distortion, the necessity of a proper recording has been felt acutely. The purpose of a case record is to keep all the information adequately and accurately recorded for future references. Case record should communicate the exact picture of the patient which has been obtained by the physician. This is possible only when recording is done properly without being hindered by any subjectivity of the physician. While giving directions for investigating the case, Master Hahnemann has greatly emphasized the necessity of being unprejudiced and stressed the need of fidelity in tracing the picture to overcome the subjectivity in practice.

Very often it is noticed that all the information of the sick person do not find a place in case record. While the physician might fail to record some information, he might unduly focus on some other. All the events and effects should be recorded without any interpolation or deletions. While recording, beginners are cautioned not to get influenced by the symptoms of drugs as recorded in the Materia Medica.

Very often the use of technical terms can create confusion, so it should be avoided, but at the same time, physician should apply common sense while noting down the picture in patient's own language. In our practice, for instance, we come across many cases where patient shows hypogastrium and says, "Doctor, I have got stomach ache." For gas (flatulence) complaints, some patients might say "I have got gastric," etc. Whatever the patient is trying to communicate should be properly received and interpreted by the physician. The physician should be careful while interpreting the words of the patient as the prejudices of the physician might crawl in here without his awareness.

Though much is said about prejudice, it is an accepted fact that remaining unprejudiced is not an easy task. Kent once stated "It would almost seem impossible to find at the present time one who could be thus described (unprejudiced)" To be unprejudiced is to be aware of our own prejudices. Once we are aware of them, the chances of committing wrong interpretations and recording them would be less.

Intensity of symptom should also be given due consideration while recording. Each and every symptom should be recorded by putting marks above it.

For example:

Salt craving 3 (more intense)

Salt craving 2 (intense)

Salt craving (moderate)

For effective repertorisation, precise recording is very crucial for proceeding further with the subsequent steps. Recording is not done independent of interpretation; so both should be done simultaneously.

DEFINITION OF PROBLEM:

Once the case is taken well, interpreted, and recorded properly the physician should be in a position to define the problem precisely. The record should guide him to understand the person and his disease. The sickness of the person gets expressed at his various levels, and to bring all such expressions together to get a whole picture, requires a clear understanding of what Hahnemann stated " what is to be cured in a disease, that is to say in every individual case of disease ".To define a problem means to define the individual who is facing the problem. The individual is fully revealed to a physician from the effects of different events associated with the individual as well as from the related data collected from various sources. Diagnosis of the disease, which is of crucial importance, would segregate the peculiar characteristic expressions from the common ones. Thus, only by precisely defining the problem, a physician would be in a position to go ahead further in the right direction.

CLASSIFICATION AND EVALUATION OF SYMPTOMS

It is a well-known fact that all the symptoms in a case are not equally important. After taking the case, a physician faces quite a big number of symptoms which are required to be analyzed, classified, and evaluated in order to arrange such symptoms hierarchically. Dr. Elizabeth Wright has given a very practical solution to this problem:" As soon as the case is taken and the physician sits down to study it, he will find it useful to run down the list of symptoms and mark with M opposite the Mentals, G opposite Generals, PATH opposite the Pathology , P opposite the particular and O for Objectives.

For further clarifying , he may under line and peculiar symptoms in red". This exercise undoubtedly is very useful for beginners, but it can prove equally beneficial to all the practitioners. However, the experienced and seasoned practitioners do it mentally.

Analysis and classification give an idea about the case in respect of its nature and the type of symptoms, and therefore, evaluation can be done by different methods.

The schema of the order of importance of symptoms according to Kent is

Mental :

Will (Emotion)

Understanding

Intellect

Physical generals :

Time, temperature, weather, position, motion, external stimuli, eating, drinking, sleep, clothing, and bathing.

Particulars :

Strange, rare and peculiar and particular modalities.

While Boger specially stresses pathological general, Boenninghausen gives more importance to concomitants and modalities. All the three evaluation methods are to help the physician, and not to confuse him. After the case is well taken, evaluation of symptoms according to the case would not be difficult. The case may have different dimensions, which may prove useful to find out the simillimum. The objective of all these methods is the same, i.e. to find out a correspondence, but case should be analyzed and evaluated by different methods and techniques to facilitate the process of finding out the simillimum.

The three standard methods of classification and evaluation propounded by Boenninghausen, Kent and Boger are of practical use in repertorisation.

ERECTING TOTALITY:

Totality is not the sum total of symptoms, but it is a logical combination of the symptoms which characterizes the person as well individualize the problem Thus, all the symptoms which are classified and evaluated do not form a working totality of the case.

From the classification and evaluation, the hierarchy of symptoms is known, but which, among them, should be useful for getting a correspondence are yet to be finalized. Thus, a physician is required to understand the whole symptom and select a few of which can logically represent the whole picture. This logical arrangement must follow a definite principle. If the case has got more generals and a few particulars with rare modalities, it would follow a different arrangement than a case which has vague modalities and striking concomitants, or a pathological general.

Totality should be erected according to the facts collected in the case. There is no hard and fast rule to erect totality in any fixed way. The case alone decides the method to be followed.

SELECTION OF REPERTORY AND REPERTORISATION PROPER:

After the totality has been erected, the case becomes clear to the physician. He should look for one of the following points in the case:

1. Generals : Mentals/Physicals.

2. Particulars: Location

Sensation

Modalities

Concomitants

3. Pathological generals.

If a case is full of generals, Kent's repertory would be the best selection. If it has got pathological general, Boger's repertory must be selected. If the case has got particulars with Location, Sensation, Modalities, Concomitants with a few mentals, therapeutic pocket book is preferable; however, Boger's repertory can also be used.

Synthetic repertory can be used for the Kent method to refer to more Generals. It has also many pathological generals, but no particulars.

Once the repertory is selected, a major part of analysis and synthesis of the case is done. The next step is to rearrange the totality according to the repertory selected. Rearrangement of the totality in terms of repertory selected is called Repertorial Totality. Thus, a well arranged totality is worked out.

What follows next is to convert the symptoms into rubrics which requires an acquaintance with the repertory. The symptoms obtained from the patient may not be found in the repertory in the same form; so the physician must know the construction and arrangement of the each repertory.

Rubrics should be arranged according to hierarchy, reason, and page number. The final out come is written as follows :

Symptoms	Rubrics	Reason	Page No.
1.	–	–	–
2.	–	–	–
3.	–	–	–

REPERTORIAL RESULT:

A group of close running medicines should be noted down according to the symptoms covered and marks obtained. For example, if Lycopodium covers seven rubrics and gets 18 marks, it should be written 18/7. A few medicines which are nearer to the first also find place in the repertorial result.

ANALSIS AND PRESCRIPTION:

The remedy which gets the highest mark is not necessarily the final remedy in all the cases. Repertorial result should be finally referred to the court of Materia Medica. Marks are important but these does not constitute the final verdict. Further the group has to be referred to the picture of the patient and with the help of Materia Medica, it should be differentiated. Sounding a note of caution, Boenninghausen writes, " for this purpose, he should not content himself with repertories that have been prepared, a very frequent carelessness for these books contain only slight hints as to one or the other remedy that might be selected but can never take the place of the careful reading up of the fountain sources". (The field which differentiates medicines is called Potential Differential Field).

Repertory, thus narrows down the group of medicines, and with the help of source books, a final remedy can be found out. The remedy so selected must finally pass through certain criteria such as susceptibility, sensibility, suppression (if any), the level of similarity, functional and structural changes, vitality, and miasm to arrive at right potency and doses schedule.

E. METHODS AND TECHNIQUES OF REPERTORISATION

For using a repertory effectively and to derive maximum benefit, one must thoroughly acquaint himself with it . Hence the need for its constant handling and frequent use.

Every repertory follows its own philosophy and construction suitable for different types of cases. Methods have been evolved as per the given philosophy underlying each repertory. Hence a case must be handled keeping in mind, first and foremost, the particular philosophy and the construction of each repertory, and not just its method.

It is commonly found that many practitioners use just one repertory for working out all cases. Such a practice is not all too desirable. Every case has its own dimension which decides the selection of repertory, and every repertory has its own methods of repertorisation.

METHODS OF REPERTORISATION:

Dr. B.K.Sarkar in his book *Lectures in Homoeopathy* (1956) has described the following methods of working out the cases:

1) Hahnemann and Boenninghausen's method = where complete symptoms are available.

2) Kent's method = Where Generals (mental and physical) and particulars are available.

3) Third method = Where mental symptoms are lacking. Here one starts with physical generals; next mental symptoms and then particulars.

4) Fourth Method = Where Generals are lacking. Selection of a striking, peculiar as a key symptom, and then medicines are differentiated with the help of other symptoms.

5) Fifth Method = Where the case presents only common symptoms or pathology. Here physician makes use of every means at his command, including

(a) Patient's personal and family history,

(b) Temperament,

(c) Complexion, color and texture of skin,

(d) Particular organs and tissues affected,

(e) Location, character and physical aspect of lesions, and

(f) Probable etiological factors.

(6) Sixth Method = Technical nosological terms are selected as main headings.

The methods described above have their own advantages and disadvantages.

TECHNIQUES OF REPERTORISATION

- Plain paper technique (old tech)
- Chart technique (New tech)
- Thumb finger technique (Artistic tech)
- Card technique
- Computer technique
- Autovisual technique
- Coin Playing technique

1. *Plain Paper Technique*
- This is also called old technique of repertorization.

- In this technique symptoms are arranged according to method of repertorization, after repertorial analysis write all the rubrics according to repertory used.

Then one by one take rubrics and write all the medicines with their proper grades. According to methods of repertorization.

- After writing down the remedies against all symptoms or rubrics, compare and count the marks and percentage of covered symptoms thus we come to the group of remedies with the knowledge of MM for final selection.

e.g. working of the following totality by Plane paper technique.

1. Abstraction of mind
2. Thirst for large quantity

Headache increases and decreases with sun.

- Abstraction of mind –

  Alum, Amel. n, Camp, *Can.i.*, Carbo.ac., Caust, Cic, Con, Cycl, Elaps, Guai, Hell, *Hyos, Kreos*, Laur, Lyc, Lyss, Mez, *Nat. m.* Nux. m, Op, Ph.ac., Phos, Plat, Sabad, Sec, Sil, Stram, *Sulph* Vesp, Visc.

- Thirst for large quantity –

  Aco, Ars, Bad, Bry, Camph, Carb. s., *Chin*, Cocc, Coc. c., Cop, *Eup. per, Fer. p.*, Ham, *Lac. d., Lycps, Merc. c*, Nat. m., Phos, Pic. ac., Sol. n, *Stram*, Sulph, Verat.

- Headache increases and decreases with sun

Aco, Glon, *Kalm*, Nat. m., Phos, Sang, Spig, Stann, Stram.

- Result of Repertorisation:

Remedies	1	2	3	4	Total
Aconite	-	2	-	1	3/2
Arsenic	-	3	2	-	5/2
Bryonia	-	3	2	-	5/2
Natrum M	2	3	2	2	9/4
Phos	3	3	-	2	8/3

- *Advantages*:
  - Byworking with this technique, one can learn repertory in better way.
  - Any piece of paper or notebook is sufficient to record the rubrics, sub rubrics ad remedies.
  - After studying and comparing rubrics and remedies ones knowledge of MM will going to increase.

- *Disadvantages*:
  - It is much time consuming and laborius than any other technique
  - Error may occur in writing remedies in exact grades and rubrics

Finding our similimum from the vast list of medicines demands good practice.

2.. CHART TECHNIQUE

- This is also called new or modern technique of repertorization but as compare to computer this is old technique of Repertorization.
- Students commonly use this technique and also one who is a new comer in the field of Homoeopathy.
- This technique is very simple and more reliable than any other technique.

- For this technique, repertorization sheet or chart is used which contains, all of the important remedies of MM printed according to alphabetical order from above downwards and the symptom numbers listed horizontally
- Working by Chart technique is done in the following way:
- Repertorization chart:

Remedy/ Symptom	1	2	3	4	5	6	7	8	9	10	11	12	Total
Aconite	3	2	-	-	3	-	-	2	2	2	1	3	18/8
Belladonna	-	3	2	-	1		3	-	2	-	2	3	17/7
Cina		-	2	3	1	-	3	2	2	-	3	-	16/7
Chamomilla	1	3	-	-	1	1	2	1	2	-	1	-	12/8
Drosera	3	2	3	2	1	-	2	-	3	2	2	3	23/10
Euphrasia	-	3	2	-	-	2	-	2	3	-	2	1	15/7

Here we have to write number of rubrics and give marks against medicine which are indicated for that rubric according to its value, leastly count the mark and select remedy according to marks obtained and symptoms covered by remedy.

- *Advantages*:
  - Only recording of remedy with grades requires less time.
  - After doping total we can easily get the similar and other auxiliary remedies
  - Easy method
  - Most reliable method.

- *Disadvantages*:
  - Repertorization sheet or chart may not be available with each and every physician

- Number of remedies recorded on the form may not have the prescribing medicine.

THUMB FINGER TECHNIQUE

- Useful in routine practice.
- This technique is used by more experienced physician who has thorough knowledge of Repertory and MM.
- It is used for quick reference.
- Physician only refers required rubrics during consultation to confirm the remedy with the knowledge of MM.
- In this technique, he uses his thumb and finger to compare different rubrics.
- No much paper work is required.

Card Technique

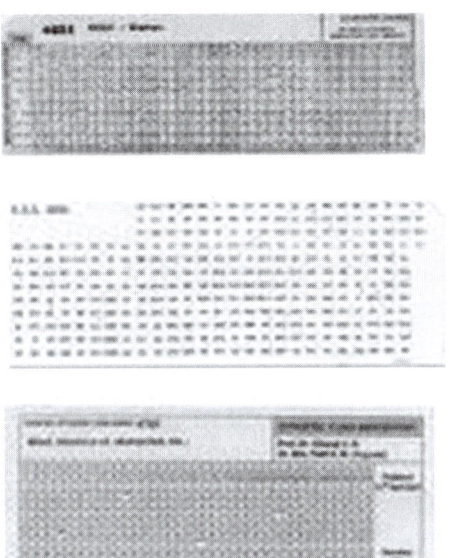
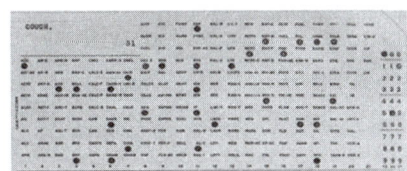
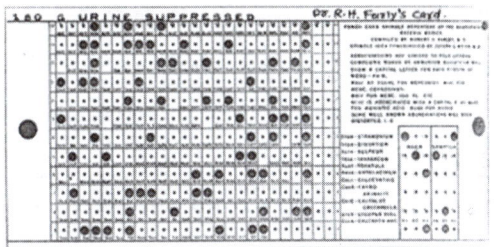

CARD TECHNIQUE

- These are actually not the repertory but it is one of the technique used for repertorization with the help of which one can repertorise very quickly.
- The card repertory possesses either, Kent Repertory, BTPB, BBCR, BSK etc.
- The Card repertory comprises of two subjects
1. The booklet
2. The Cards
- The booklet comprises the lists of rubrics particularly with their serial number or code numbers and also philosophical background and the process of working with illustrations
- The cards though are of various kinds, but mainly contain either the names of the medicines enlisted in alphabetical manner or the code numbers of the medicines. Punching or holes are made under the code numbers which become the indicated remedy for the very rubric which is generally recorded on the top of the card with their code numbers.
- When the card has been selected according to the rubric and placed one above the other, we can see the light passing through the holes.
- The holes from which the light passes, we have to consider the code number of that medicine and select the final medicine with the help of booklet.
- Advantages and Disadvantages wide separately in the topic of card repertory.

COMPUTER TECHNIQUE

- In this technique, different softwares are made and repertories are uploaded in it.

- The technique is same as we do in chart technique. The only difference is that the written work we do in chart technique is minimized with the help of computer.

- In this technique, after making a repertorial totality, we have to select the rubric by clicking the button and after selecting all rubrics with the help of just one click we get the group of remedies.

- Advantages and Disadvantages wide separately in the topic of computer repertory.

AUTOVISUAL TECHNIQUE

- This is actually not the repertory but it is one of the technique used for repertorization with the help of which one can repertorise very quickly.

- It consists of
  1. Autostrips
  2. Autovisual apparatus
  3. Booklet

1. Autostrips:

- All autostrips have number on top representing rubric number and are grooved at several places.

- Each groove represents corresponding medicine in autovisual apparatus.

- These grooves are in different colours or markings which indicate gradation. Red = 3, Yellow=2, and Black =1

- Again there are two heavy grooves (Green) one at the top and the other at the bottom of the autostrip as "Guide lines" to match with the "Guide lines" of AV apparatus.

- The number written on the top of autostrips are also coloured some are red and some are black at the top.

General symptom's autostrips are red and particular symptom's autostrips are black.

Technique: After making repertorial totality, refer the selected rubric in the booklet with their code numbers.

Then autostrips numbers representing the selected rubrics are taken out from the autostrip box.

Arrange the rubrics numbers in the order of importance.

Fed the autostrips from the top of the apparatus one by one in order in the AV apparatus from right to left, one beside the other.

See the autostrips "Guide lines" (Green) at the top and bottom come exactly I the line with the "Guide lines" (green) in the apparatus.

The apparatus has a space to filled only ten autostrips.

The common medicine in all with highest score is one which is indicated.

Look for single straight horizontal line.

- If more than one horizontal line is obtained, these are competing remedies which match all the rubrics.

- Count the total grades by the colours in the grooves of the strips.

- You will thus get the total matchings and total grades of the medicines.

- If there is gap in the line, consider the longest lines and count the total matchings and its total grades.

- Then analyses or go to the MM for final selection.

COIN PLAYING TECHNIQUE

- It is economic, time saving enjoyable play and work for finding out the correct prescription by Arithmetic calculation. By this process one can repertorise as many cases as he likes by a single set.

- It consists of
  1. Card Board
  2. Coin

1. On the card board, different medicines are written in the respective columns. On the corner of the board

2. The coins are in four colours, Red for 5 and 3 marks, blue for 4 and 2 marks, Green for 3 and 1 marks and black for 2 marks

3. Technique –

1. Take a small piece of paper on which note down the rubrics and their pg no. of the Repertory book that you will use.

2. Read the rubrics and the medicines and place the coins in the specified rooms.

3. Lastly look for highest peaks and identify them.

4. Count the number of coins in highest peaks, total matchings and count their total values.

5. Analyse or go to MM. Enjoy repertory s a game to play

F. SALIENT FEATURES OF COMMON REPERTORIES AND THEIR UTILITY

Repertory is just a tool, it is the mind which uses it that performs the exercise. The logic of Repertories, their usage, their scope should be imbibed before working with them. So here, we discuss with you the salient features of the common Repertories and their utility:

Year	Name of Repertory	Author	No. of Remedies	No. of Pages & Chapters	Gradation in Chapters
1805	Fragmenta de viribus medica mentorum positivis sive in sano corpore humano observatis	Samuel Hahnemann	27	713 pages: (including 470 paged Alphabetical Repertory)	Single grade
1817	Symptom Dictionary (handwritten)	Samuel Hahnemann		symptoms from his materia medica.	
1826	Systematic Representation of the Pure Effects of Medicines for the Practical Use of Homeopathic Physicians	Carl George Christian Hartlaub			
1830	Systematic Description of Antipsoric Remedies	George Adolph Weber	1830		
1830-1831	Systematic Presentation of all Homeopathic Medicines, 1st manuscript not published 2nd edition: 1835	Ernst Ferdinand Ruckert		Re-arranged Hahnemann's dictionary published in three volumes.	
1832	Repertory of Antipsoric Remedies (German) 2nd Edition: 1833 English Translation - 1900 (Boger)	Clemens Franz Maria von Boenning hausen	52	44 chapts 256 pgs	**CAPITAL** **BOLD** **Roman** **Bold** *Italics* Roman Roman in parenthesis

1833	Repertory of Intermittent Fever	Clemens Franz Maria von Boenninghausen	4		Single grade
1834	Jahr's Manual of Homeopathic Medicines - 1st edition published (German) - 1841 - A Gerald Hull re-translated, revised and re-edited the New Manual of Homeopathic Medicine, became known simply as *Hull's Jahr.* - 4th edition - 1851- Boenninghausen's gradation of remedies incorporated. - 1853 - Charles J. Hempel edited - Jahr's New Manual or Symptom Encordex and the third volume the Repertory. - 1853 - with additions from Possart's work and was further revised and translated by Hempel.	George Heinrich Gottlieb Jahr		29 in 3rd edition	Single grade. In 4th edition he adopted Boenninghausen's gradation.
1835	Repertory of Medicines which are not Antipsoric - Prefaced by Hahnemann. - English Translation - Boger (1900)	Clemens Franz Maria von Boenning hausen		266 pages	

1836	An Attempt at Showing the Relative Kinship of Homeo-pathic Medicines.	Clemens Franz Maria von Boenning hausen			
1838	Repertory to Jahr's Manual published in Allentown Academy - The first repertory in English language. - Precursor of Kent's Repertory	Constantine Hering		419 pages	
1842	Pure Symptomatology or Synoptic Pattern of All The Materia medica - first Repertory in French	P.J.Lafitte, Paris		974 pages	
1846	Therapeutic Manual for Homeopathic physicians for use at the sickbed and the study of the Materia Medica Pura (Therapeutic Pocket Book) **Translators:** - In 1848, German to English translation was done by Stapf. - Boenninghausen himself did French translation. - Roth translated again German to French. - A. Harward Okie-1847 - Charles J. Hempel-1847	Clemens Franz Maria von Boenning-hausen	342	7	**CAPITAL** **BOLD** **Roman** **Bold** *Italics* Roman Roman in parenthesis

	- Laurie translated from Roth's French edition to English language. - T.F. Allen in 1891 - Added 220 remedies by dropping 4 remedies and so total 342 and incorporated *Sides of the Body*. And in Relationship of Remedies section he added 21 remedies, so altogether 142 remedies. - H.A. Roberts - Few changes with addition of few remedies (18 remedies) and a beautiful introduction given to the Therapeutic Pocket Book - 1935. - Recent revised edition by Gypser and Dimitriadis - 2000.			
1848	Manual of Homeo-pathic Materia medica in 3 volumes, where the 3rd volume is repertory and was later revised by Clotar Muller.	Karl Friedrich Trinks		
1851	A Pocket Manual-popular book for physicians and as 'domestic manual' for laypersons.	Joel Byrant	352 pages	

1854	The Sides of the Body and Drug Affinities.	Clemens Franz Maria von Boenning-hausen	129		4 Grades in Sides of the Body. 3 Grades in Drug Affinities.
1859	Repertory of Homeo-pathic Materia medica (Cypher Repertory) -Boger described as 'pure gold'	Robert Ellis Dudgeon		2 vol. bound as one (1878)	
1869	Homeopathic Therapeutics of Diarrhoea.	James B. Bell	141	5	**Roman** **Bold** *Italics* Roman Roman in parenthesis
1873	Complete Repertory to the Homeopathic Materia Medica, Diseases of Eyes.	E.W. Berridge	1171	2321 pages	*CAPITAL* *ITALICS* *Italics* Roman Roman in parenthesis
1875	Analytical Therapeutics -Re-issued in 1881 as Analytical Repertory of Symptoms of Mind	Constantine Hering		48, 352 pages	Boenning hausen's grades I, II, **I, II**
1879	Repertory to the More Characteristic Symptoms of the Materia Medica - Based on Hering's Allentown Repertory	Constantine Lippe	301	34, 112 pages	*Italics* Roman

1879	The Therapeutics of Intermittent Fever	Henry Clay Allen	147	9	Roman **Bold** *Italics* Roman Roman in parenthesis
1879	A Repertory of Headaches	John C. King		297 pages	
1880	Symptom Register. -Volume 11 and 12 of Allen's work	Timothy Field Allen	820	1331 pages	CAPITAL *Italics* Roman
1881	Analytical Repertory of the Symptoms of the Mind.	Constantine Hering	669	48	4 grades: I, II, **I, II**
1882	The Homeopathic Therapeutics of Haemorrhoids.	W.M. Jefferson Guernsey	135	3	Roman **Bold** *Italics* Roman
1885	Alphabetical Repertory - First in India	Father Muller			
1889	Guernsey's Boenning hausen Slips.	W.J. Guernsey	126	2500 cards	Boenning hausen's 4 grades
1890	The Concordance Repertory of the More Characteristic Symptoms of the Materia Medica	William D. Gentry	420	6 volumes, 5500 pages	Single grade
1892	Ophthalmic Diseases and Therapeutics.	A. B. Norton	151	17	Single grade
1894	Sensation As If.	A. W. Holocomb			
1896	Repertory of Hering's Guiding Symptom of Our Materia Medica.	Calvin B. Knerr	408	48	4 grades: I, II, **I, II**
1897	Repertory of the Homeopathic Materia Medica	James Tyler Kent	648 - 6 = 642	37	Roman **Bold** *Italics*

	- 2nd edition: 1908 - 3rd edition: 1924 (Kent's life ended with this edition) - 4th edition: 1935 - 5th edition: 1945 - 6th edition: 1957				Roman
1898	Repertory of the Symptoms of Rheumatism, Sciatica, etc.	Alfred Pulford		28	CAPITAL *Italics* Roman
1900	A Repertory of the Cyclopaedia of Drug Pathogenesy.	Richard Hughes	412	12	Single grade
1904	A Clinical Repertory.	John Henry Clarke	994	5 parts	Single Repertory; 5 repertories have been included.
1905	Boenninghausen's Characteristics and Repertory. 2nd edition: 1937 by Roy and Co., Calcutta.	Cyrus Maxwell Boger	448	49	5 grades **CAPITAL** **BOLD** **Roman** **Bold** *Italics* Roman Roman in parenthesis
1906	Boericke's Repertory - 3rd edition onwards the repertory part was incorporated though the first edition came in 1901.	Oscar Eugene Boericke	1405	25	*Italics* Roman
1922	Fields Card Repertory (Symptom Register)	Richard Field	360	6800 cards	1st and 2nd grade of Kent's Repertory

1926	The General Analysis - printed form.	Cyrus Maxwell Boger	222		Single grade
1928	The General Analysis - Card Repertory.	Cyrus Maxwell Boger	22	304 cards	Single 2 grade
1931	Synoptic Key to the Materia Medica.	Cyrus Maxwell Boger	323	4	3 grades CAPITAL **Roman Bold** Ordinary Roman
1932	Addition's to Kent's Repertory	Cyrus Maxwell Boger		37	CAPITAL *Italics* Roman Roman in parenthesis
1937	Sensation As If - A Repertory of Subjective Symptoms.	Herbert A. Roberts	740	25	Single grade
1937	Times of Remedies and Moon Phases. Boger	Cyrus Maxwell	330 186	9 4	3 grades Single grade
1939	Unabridged Dictionary of the Sensation As If.	James William Ward		2 volumes	Single grade
1939	Repertory to the Rheumatic Remedies.	Herbert A. Roberts	207	25	CAPITAL SMALL CAPITALS *Italics* Roman
1948	Practical Homeo-pathic Repertory in colored and perforated cards - Gradation of drugs.	Marcos Jimenez	480	552 cards	3 grades. Red Sq. Blue Sq. Uncolored Square
1950	Spindle's Card Repertory	Robert H. farley	274	190 cards	

1959	Kishore's Card Repertory	Jugal Kishore	692 in 3rd ed.	9192 cards	Single card
1963	A Concise Repertory of Homeopathic Med. - 2nd Edition: 1977	S. R. Phatak		Alphabetical	CAPITAL *Italics* Roman
1972	Synthetic Repertory	Barthel and Klunker	1594	3 volumes	**<u>BOLD CAPITAL -UNDERLINE</u>** **BOLD CAPITAL** **Small Letter Bold** Small letter
1974	Additions to Kent's Repertory	George Vithoulkas			Same as that of Kent
1978	A Handbook of Repertory	Major K. K. Sirkar		41	**Bold** *Italics* Roman
1980	The Final General Repertory	Diwan Harish Chand and Pierre Schmidt			
1981	Sequelae	G. S. R. Sastry			
1984	Sharma's Card Repertory	Shashi Mohan Sharma	400	3000 cards	
1987	Repertorium Generale	Jost Kunzlli von Fimmelsberg	682	37	**Bold** **Roman** *Italics* Roman
1990	Alphabetical Repertory of Characteristics of Homeopathic Materia Medica	G. D. Srivastava and J. Chandra	680	Alphabetical	Single grade
1993	Synthesis Repertorium Homoeopathicum Syntheticum	Frederik Schroyens	2373	38	**CAPITAL** **BOLD** **Bold** **Roman** *Italics* Roman

1993	Homeopathic Medical Repertory -2nd Edition - 1997	Robin Murphy	1595	70	**CAPITAL** **BOLD** *Italics* Roman
1995	Thematic Repertory	J. A. Mirrili			
1996	Complete Repertory	Roger Van Zandvoort	1725	42	**BOLD** **CAPITAL** **<u>UNDERLINE</u>** CAPITAL ***Bold Italics*** Roman
1999	The Phoenix Repertory	J. P. S. Bakshi	1225	38	**BOLD** **CAPITAL** **<u>-UNDERLINE</u>** CAPITAL ***Bold Italics*** Roman
2005	Repertorium Universalis	Roger Van Zandvoort		43	**BOLD** **CAPITAL** **<u>UNDERLINE</u>** CAPITAL ***Bold Italics*** Roman

G. CLASSIFICATION OF REPERTORIES

The number of repertories available in the market has increased manifolds since the time of master Hahnemann. There are about 200 various types of repertories which can be helpful for different purposes.

Purpose of classification

Each classified group is a representative of specific application and value Grouping will help to highlights the group characteristics and individual peculiarities of the repertories.

The classification is necessary to group the similar repertories together ,so when the schools of philosophy points to a group of repertories ,the most similar among can be selected for repertorisation.

Levels of classification

- Overall appearance
- Internal formatting
- Group characteristics

LEVEL.1 OVER ALL APPEARANCES

- Book Repertories
- Card Repertories
- Software Packages

Book repertories

Most of the repertories are available in the book form.

Advantage

They are most numerous and easily available

They are cost effective

They are easy to carry and to use

Disadvantage

Due to multiplicity very difficult to select the required repertory.

Up gradation & Corrections are difficult

Out dated terminologies are used in many repertories.

Card repertories

Is a system of visual sorting which eliminate the necessarily of righting out the rubrics & remedies against them. Even though it has many advantages they are outdated in the event of computers.

Computer repertories

They have many appealing features. The number of options available for reference is immense and the work is also very fast, may also carried to the bedside in the form of laptop computers.

LEVEL. 2 INTERNAL FORMATTING

Based on the internal formatting they are divided in to

- Puritan group
- Logical utilitarian group

Puritan group – They are called so because the purity of the language of the drug proving is maintained. They are used for the purpose of reference and not for systemic repertorisation. They help us to refer the symptoms without much variations in the language of the provers. Thes repertories are analogues to the index of the symptoms as they are presented in the materia medica.

Kneer repertory

Gentry's repertory

Logical utilitarian group – are called so because of their arrangement and their utility value, they have distinct principles of their own.

In this repertories the symptoms may not be found in the language of the materiamedica, but the symptoms change their forms to fit in to the arrangement of the repertories.

Eg. Kent's repertory

Synthesis.

LEVEL. 3 GROUP CHARACTERISTICS

The classification made on the basis of group characteristics is the most pragmatic one for selecting the repertory according to the demands of the case.

1. **General repertories**

    Based on deductive logic

    E.g. Kent's repertory

    Based on inductive logic

    E.g. Therapeutic pocket book

    Based on Clinical approach

    E.g. Repertory to Homoeopathic MM by Oscar E Boericke

2. **Regional repertories**

    Dealing with the organs

    E.g. Berridges Repertory to Eye Dealing with the system

    E.g. Morgan's repertory to urinary organs

3. **Particular repertories**

    Dealing with particular states

    Eg. Repertory to time modalities

    Dealing with the particular diseased condition

    Eg. Repertory of diarrhoea By Bell James

4. **Alphabetical repertories**

    The symptoms are arranged in alphabetical order

    Eg. Repertory to Homoeopathic MM By Pathak

5. **Concordance repertories**

    Repertory of Concordance by Kneer

6. **Comparative repertories**

    Comparative repertory of Hom.MM by Docks & Kockelenberg

7. **Pathogenic repertory**

    Repertory to Cyclopedia of drug pathogenesy by Richard Huges

8. **Reference repertories**

    Select your remedy by Biswamber das

9. **Therapeutic digests**

    Raue's special pathology & therapeutics

10. **Card repertories**
    Kishore's cards

11. **Computer repertories**
    CARA, RADAR, HOMPATH

1.   GENERAL REPERTORIES

The general repertories are logical utilitarian repertories.

Useful for individualization as desired by the principles of Homoeopathy.

They facilitate the adapt ion of general symptom for repertorisation.

3 major groups

a. **Based on deductive logic**

    Here the generals are given prime importance, then follows characteristics particulars. The analysis of the case for these repertories is also based on the premise of the deductive logic, where the generals symptoms are given higher ranking than the particular symptoms.

E.g. Kent's repertory, Synthesis

Synthetic repertory also adopted the principles of deductive logic but do not included particular symptoms.

b. **Based on inductive logic**

Means from particulars to generals

In these repertories the different elements of a symptom like location sensation modality & concomitants can be brought together on the basis of certain constants & and a general symptom can be constructed .The resulting general symptom is called a Synthetic general.

When there is a particular sensation that is expressed at more than two location at any given time, the sensation can be elevated to the level of a general symptom, provided the modalities remain the same for all the locations expressing that sensation. If a concomitant is also present the generalization become stronger.

E.g. TPB is based on doctrine of analogy & concomitant Boger's repertory operates on complete symptom Synoptic key by Boger give important to pathological generals.

c. **Clinical repertories**

These repertories have many clinical rubrics under different systems, and the medicines are given against the name of the disease.

As in the general repertories the clinical repertories also cover the therapeutic information for the whole of the organism & come under logical utilitarian group.

The construction of these repertories affords the flexibility of adopting either the deductive or inductive logic at any given time, and highly useful when there is a significant amount of clinical data available in a case.

Eg. Clinical repertory by J.H.Clark

The prescriber by J.H.Clark

2. **REGIONAL REPERTORIES**

Regional repertories mainly focus on the information relevant to a particular system or a region. They are mainly used for reference purposes, not for individualisation, but having the advantage of elaborating on a particular theme witha high degree of specificity.

Eg. Berridg's eye

Morgan's urinary organs

3. **PARTICULAR REPERTORIES**

These repertories are based on clinical orientation, focused on certain particular states or particular diseased condition. The specific state may be a modifying factor. This repertories also affords a high degree of specification in the particular area.

E.g. Time modalities by Shedd.P.V

Diarrhoea by Bell james

4. **ALPHABETICAL REPERTORIES**

The symptoms in this repertories are arranged in a alphabetical order. This repertories are qualifying as general repertories to a reference book.

Eg. General alphabetical repertories

Murphy's repertory

Pathak repertory

Clinical alphabetical repertories

The presciber by Clark

Reference repertories

Highlights of Homoeopathic practice by T.P.Chatterjee

5. CONCORDANCE REPERTORIES

Word meaning In agreement or In harmony

OR

An index of words or passages of a book or an author

Here the medicine is analyzed for its relationship with other medicines at different levels and at different spheres. Logical utilitarian repertories are popular as repertories and the puritan repertories are known as Concordance repertories or Concordances.

These repertories are comprised of mainly of the symptoms in the language of the provers, the whole symptoms expressed by the patient may be obtained as a single unit in these books. The demerit is that the search is very difficult & time consuming.

6. COMPARATIVE REPERTORIS

This is one of the latest repertories, which is aimed to assist the user in differentiating the medicines with in the rubric, often this save the labor of consulting the materia medica for the differential references.

This repertory is a beginning of a movement for improving the service of repertory use. The comparative repertory is deficient in data, because all the remedies are not compared and differentiated.

E.g. Comparative repertory by Docks & Kockelenberg.

7. PATHOGENIC REPERTORIES

This is an index to the symptoms as presented during the drug proving. This repertory is useful when the pathological changes form the only available database in a case. Also useful in case where the differentiation of the medicines and prescription of the appropriate remedy has to be made only on the basis of the objective symptoms.

In concordance repertories the symptoms are written in the language of the provers _ the verbal expression. But in the pathogenic repertories the expression at the level of altered physiological phenomena & the pathological process are explained.

E.g. Repertory of drug pathogenesy By Richard Huges.

8. REFERENCE REPERTORIES

These are not repertories in strict sense, but these books are handy for prescribing in acute cases and in cases with insufficient data.

They are used as ready recokners for assessing the information about a symptom or a condition with certain constant features.

E.g. Qiuck bed side presciber by Singhal.

9. THERAPEUTIC DIGESTS

These are miniature versions of repertories and deals mainly with a particular clinical condition.

E.g. Raue's Special pathology & therapeutic hints.

H. ADVANTAGES AND LIMITATIONS OF REPETORY

Repertory is an index of homoeopathic materia medica which is full of information collected from toxicology, drug proving and clinical experiences.

The process of **repertorisation** is essentially an elimination, which starts with a broad choice and slowly narrows down the field, giving us adequate small group of medicine, so that the final selection is made easier with the help of further reference to the materia medica.

The physician who have never used or have rarely used repertory complains about its elaborate methods and time consuming nature, but one who has used it meaningfully find it is highly useful and time saving.

1. **To avoid routinism**

   For a stomach pain ameliorated by hard pressure a routine prescriber settles his prescription upon Bryonia, but in repertory under Stomach – pain-pressure ameliorate, there are 7 remedies but no Bryonia. Repertory teaches the physician to be careful in the selection of the medicine and avoid routionism.

2. **It teaches** by gradation the relative importance of various medicines.
   It is important that symptoms according to their intensity [gradation] in a patient must match with similar intensity in the medicine chosen. An ideal homoeopath make an analysis of each symptom in each case and make the final selection according to the intensity and gradation of each symptom of the patient as found in the medicine.

3. **To select similimum quickly**.
   Repertory reduces the laborious work of repertorising the whole case, when there is peculiar and striking symptoms or if their is any etiology which can be referred in the appropriate repertory immediately. So repertory simplifies and strengthens our selection for particular medicine.

4. **Helps to find out complete symptom.**
   In repertory, a complete symptom with all its components can be referred to one place, especially concomitance which are scattered in several places in materia medica.

5. **It promote discovery of medicine.**
   which one had not thought of. such symptom would remain in his mind forever.

6. **Second prescription.**
   It suggest related remedies which could be helpful for selecting a drug for follow up or second prescription.

7. **Its constant use makes the physician efficient.**
   By constant handling one refreshes the knowledge of M.M, difficult symptoms and medicines with different grades.

8.. **It help the physician to ask intelligent questions.**

Some times the patients are not able to tell their symptoms correctly or the physician not able to get the symptoms from them for the choice of medicine ,under such circumstances one can use repertory to his advantage and finally chose the medicine by asking questions guided by repertory.

9. **Repertory teaches us** to be careful about those symptoms belonging to the disease [common symptoms] and to consider only those symptoms which lie outside the disease [uncommon symptoms of the disease].

Allopaths diagnose the disease for the purpose of commencing the treatment where as homoeopaths diagnose the disease for the purpose of removing the common symptom of the disease and to consider the rest of the symptom that lie outside the path gnomonic symptom.

Repertory makes the study of M.M extremely interesting and revels more and more about uncommon symptoms. When we are in doubt a rubric, the meaning of which is not clear, we are compelled to read the materia medica for the exact meaning.

10. **It help the study of Materia medica.**

Take any drug and refer any section in the repertory which one wants to study and not down the presence of remedy against the given rubric.

Help in comparative study of drugs.

The intensity of symptom in a drug can be studied which help in the final selection of medicine.

Repertory expand our knowledge by giving more remedies for keynotes.

11. **To recall.**

Sometimes a symptom strikes a physican, but unable to recall the medicine. In such cases he can seek the help of repertory.

12. **To find out the similimum.**

Symptoms are converted in to rubrics, these rubrics are located in the repertory. The repertory gives an idea about co running medicines, so the indicted medicine can be found out.

LIMITATIONS OF REPERTORY

- Repertoryis basically an index, never suggest a final choice.

- Different repertories have different philosophy and construction.

- New additions to materiamedica cannot be accommodated in repertory.

- Many rubrics are not represented well.

- No guidance about potency, dose and repetition.

- Nosodes and sarcodes not represented well.

- If the physician makes mistakes in interpretation, and just counting the symptoms and marks.

- Use of repertory cannot be independent of knowledge of materia medica, organon or clinical subjects.

I. RELATION BETWEEN HOMOEOPATHIC MATERIA MEDICA, ORGANON AND REPERTORY

Homoeopathic Materia Medica, Organon and repertory is a three legged stool to represent Homoeopathic System of medicine.

Dr.Kent has said, "The physician must study the homoeopathic principles until he learns what it is in sickness that guides to the curative remedy.

Dr.J.H.Clarke says, " It is impossible to practice Homoeopathy without the aid of repertories".

Repertory is a ' tool' appropriate tool is necessary to carry out a specific job like a good artisan, we must be familiar with all types of tools - their utility and limitations.

Homoeopathy is based on the Law of Similars. Homoeopathic Physician, in his attempt to Cure, constantly attempts to establish similarity between the two phenomena :

1) The artificial drug disease recorded in the Hom. Mat. Medica and

2) The natural disease - recorded in the case Record

The similarity between the two phenomena is to be established at the conceptual level

viz. At the level of ' Portrait of Disease ' as Enunciated by Hahnemann

The conceptual image as it is called is based on ' Totality of Symptoms '. This

Totality is in a sense 'qualitative expression'of the disease rather than sum total of its Symptomatology.

Since it is an expression of ' qualitative' Image it has to be highly individualised

both in the case of sickness and also in the case of the drug. Individualisation is the corner stone of the homoeopathic treatment.Homoeopath studies both these phenomena keeping this central point in mind. He, therefore constantly compares and contrasts the characteristic signs and symptoms of both till he perceives the similarity between the two. In this process he evaluates all the manifestations and ascribe relative values or importance to these manifestations.

Totality of symptoms

" Every deviation from the original state of Health enjoyed by the patient "

- Deviations experienced by him
- Deviations observed by his close relatives and friends
- Deviations observed by the physician
- Any additional information gathered by the physician based on other investigations

Totality essentially qualitative and not quantitative or numerical

- Essential Characteristics of sickness
- Manner of evolution Speed, Direction, Mode and variation
- Characteristic pattern of attributes of Sick

Homoepathy is from beginning to the end, is an art of individualisation. We have to inividualise patients and individualise Remedies.

Evaluation of Symptoms

It is an exercise of giving relative value (not absolute value) to different signs and symptoms of the patient.

It is necessary for the purpose of building a portrait of the sick person out of his symptoms and this process is called as SYNTHESIS.

Repertory is a tool

Appropriate tool is necessary to carry out a specific job. Like a good artisan, we must be familiar with all types of tools their utility and limitations.

The disease to be perceived in -

- Perversion of desires and aversions
- Perversion of intellect
- Disturbed memory
- Perverted physical sensations
- Disturbed function of system/organ with attending modalities
- Perverted sensations and suffering of parts

- Tissue changes and pathological conditions
- Causes that excite each of these are parallel
- To the perverted states themselves in each sphere.

General principles of repertorisation

- Totality
- Causation
- Generalisation
- Individualization
- Analysis of the Case
- Evaluation of the symptomatology
- Synthesis or ' Portrait ' building

The material medica is an ocean full of medicines and symptoms and a suitable tool is required to find the right medicine at right time. The organon guides us how to make the best use of these medicines with appropriate principles.

J. LOGIC

INTRODUCTION:

Logic is a Greek word, which means Discourse. When we try to understand the word Discourse it suggest that it is a communication of ideas, information etc. The study of logic began in ancient Greece. Whenever man debates, discuss, and argue logic remains in the background. Whenever a man debates a matter in his own mind a silent logic plays role. No man can think without logic. If he will try to break logic will break him. Logic has created deep and long lasting impression on language and culture. Logic is the air, which we breathe. It is a connected thought expressed in words. Discourse with one self is called meditation. From what others have said or from what we ourselves have thought conclusions and inferences are drawn. They are the special concern of logic. Logic trains the mind to draw right conclusion and to avoid wrong. It always deals with serious statement.

Definition: From Aristotle to Mill several definitions of Logic have been suggested. Each and every definition is unique. They are closely related to each other.

According to oxford dictionary: "Logic is a science of reasoning."

Discussion of definition: On the basis of above-mentioned definition it is necessary for us to know the relation between science and reasoning. The word reasoning indicates: "The drawing of inferences or conclusions from known or assumed facts." If we want to represent any of our concept it is necessary that it must be based on sound explanation of Philosophy and it must be verified by scientific experiments. Such Philosophical argument, which is supported by scientific experiments, is nothing but Logic. So we can say that Logic is a beautiful coordination of Science and Philosophy. Unless a person knows science and philosophy deeply he will not able to reason any thing. No doubt he will have that power of doing argument but it will not consider as logical.

Relation between Science and Philosophy: According to Funk and Wan galls dictionary science in the widest sense includes: exact knowledge of facts, exact knowledge of laws obtained by correlation of facts, exact knowledge of proximate causes.

Philosophy is the general principle, laws, or causes that furnished the rational explanation of anything. Science and Philosophy are not antagonist but they are complementary to each other. Philosophy is a hypothetical interpretation. Science arises in hypothesis and flows in to interpretation. Science is descriptive but it divides one thing in to many sub categories. Like organs, parts of body, diseases, etc. philosophy is the criticism of categories. Science describes philosophy while philosophy teaches us to accept science. Every science begins as philosophy and ends as an art. If we want to develop the art of reasoning we must develop the art of thinking, perceiving, and proper interpreting. Reasoning is the minds eye.

If we want to develop the power of reasoning we make the habit of reading in between the lines. Reading enables us to explain the different phenomena critically. It is the intellectual faculty by which conclusions are drawn from premises by connected thoughts. It teaches us how one judgment arrives from other judgment. Any process of inference is based on reasoning. **So logic is called science of inference.** It provides us light in the dark way of searching truth.

History related to origin of Logic: The demand for logic aroused in ancient Greece from the Sophistic movement. Sophists were pioneers of higher education. As a result there were disputes so they required rules for regulating discussion. Logic supplied the rules. Aristotle was one of the greatest thinkers of all time and he wrote on logic which includes:

Prior analytic. [Formal aspect of Syllogistic reasoning.]

Posterior analytics. [Deeper problems of inference.]

Concept of various stalwarts related to logic:

1. **Concept of Aristotle:** Aristotle is considering as the founder of true logic because he systematically arranged different methodologies of logic and he is the father of both deductive and inductive logic. The most important logical work of Aristotle was organon. His method of logic was based on "Syllogism". It is a Greek word. The meaning of this word is reasoning in general.

2. **Concept of Lord Francis Bacon** [1561-1626]:

   His life: He was associated with royal family of England. He left the Cambridge school by saying that these studies are useless. In 1618 Lord Chancellor arrested for taking bribes but queen pardoned him but he had to abandon public life. He is considering as founder of modern inductive logic and said it is the only method of scientific discovery. He also introduced logical systematization of scientific procedures. His two important major writings are:

   1. Advancement of learning.

   2. Novum Organum

   According to Bacon there are two ways of investigating and discovering the truth.

   1. Inductive Logic.

   2. Deductive Logic.

1. **Inductive Logic:**

a. **Introduction**: The Inductive method in science is the application of the principles of inductive logic to scientific research. Lord Bacon originated this method. He set forth in his Novum Organum. John Stuart mill in his great System of Logic further developed it. It has been the inspiration, the basis and the instrument of every modern science.

b. **Dictionary Meaning**: The word has originated from the word Induce that means to tell someone to do something or to cause something to happen. The word induction suggests:

   1. Logical Reasoning.

   2. The process of being initiated.

---

c. **Definition**: "Inductive method in logic is the scientific method that proceeds by Induction."

"Induction is a process of drawing universal conclusion from Particular premise."

d. **Basic Characteristics of Inductive Logic**: The way of argument of this logic is rested on principles a posteria. This indicates that in this method principles are derived from our uncontradicated experience. In other words we can say that we accept it without contradiction. On the base of these arguments we never yields a necessary truth. This does not indicate that Inductive Logic is only a wild speculation. But in this method of logic conclusion does not necessarily follow from it premises. This condition is seen in deductive method of logic. Here conclusion is based on a certain degree of probability. Greater the reliability of premises higher the probability of the truth of conclusion.

Here particular conclusion is drawn from particular to general. For example: Tom, Hick, Harry have yellow eyes. They have Jaundice. Therefore those who all have yellow eyes have Jaundice. Here it is noticeable that the transition here is from the part to the whole from the particular to universal from some particular truth we leap to generalized truth.

By inductive reasoning we ascertain what is true of many different things. Our senses tell us what happens around us and by proper reasoning we may discover the laws of nature, in consequence of which they happen.

Every mind conceives intuitively some ideas or judgments which are at once primary and certain otherwise we could have no foundation for inference and to infer one idea or judgment from others would give no certainty. These ideas are called first truths. They are given by the senses, the consciousness and the reason and they are innumerable. For example: "I exist. There is an external world. This body is solid, extended, round, red, warm or cold are first truths." At first these ideas are particular but afterward the mind unites those which are similar or which agree in some respect in to classes. This is called "Generalization". To express this we no longer say this or that body but body, not coat, shirt, trousers, but clothes only.

2. **Deductive Logic:**

a. **Introduction:** The deductive method in science is the application of the principles of deductive logic to scientific research.

b. **Dictionary Meaning**: The word has originated from the word deduce that means to

   1. Trace the course or derivation of.
   2. To infer by logical reasoning.
   3. Conclude from known facts or general principles.

The dictionary meaning of the word deduction suggests:

1. A deducting or being deducted; subtraction
2. A sum or amount deducted or allowed to be deducted.

---

c. **Definition**: "Deductive method in logic is the scientific method that proceeds by deduction."

d. **Basic Characteristics of Deductive Logic:** This method of logic works on certain basic priority principles. This method finally reach to such truths that are justified by pure thoughts or reasoning. The theme of this method is: In a valid argument if premises are true than conclusion from these premises must necessarily be true also. In this method conclusion of a deductive argument never goes beyond what the premises state. In this method conclusion is drawn from general to particular. This can be beautifully understood by example:

1. All doctors are wise. [General]
2. Kent is a doctor. [Particular]

Therefore Kent is also wise. [General To Particular.]

This is a syllogistic argument. It is a process of reasoning from out of two statements having common part. On the basis of this third statement is given. In above-mentioned example 'Doctor' is a common part, which is there in both the statements on the basis of this third statement, is given.

Logic plays important role in construction of repertories and their philosophies.

K. IMPORTANT TERMINOLOGIES IN REPERTORIES

Important terminologies in repertories:

There are few common terms in repertory which are as follows:-

- Language of the repertory
- Rubrics
- Sub rubrics
- Symptoms Vs Rubrics
- Cross Reference
- Repertorial Totality
- Potential difference field
- Hunting of rubrics
- Synthesis of rubric
- Gradation of remedy
- Repertorial Analysis
- Repertorial Result Analysis
- Generalization
- Particularization
- Repertorization

1) **LANGUAGE OF REPERTORY:** The language of the repertory is different from the language of the MM and different from the language of the patient because the repertory uses a more limited vocabulary.

   - Patients may use different words and descriptions to express the same thing.
   - This richness must be translated in the exact wording of the MM.
   - The core of the expressed symptoms or idea will be found in one way in the repertory.
   - Otherwise, consulting the repertory becomes a laborious task.

- For each symptom, we would have to think of all possible synonym and similar ways of expressing the same thing before we know all corresponding remedies.

2) **RUBRICS: HEADING/GUIDING RULE:**

A) Origin: The word rubric is originated from the Latin word *"Rubrica"* which means Heading or Guiding rule, so Rubric is a term applied to each Heading or main heading of symptoms with list of larger no. of medicines which is followed by sub rubrics.

   - In case of concordance repertories rubric is not repertorial language but this is explained in prover's language.

B) Definition: Rubrics are the repertorial language in which a big sentence is expressed by few words, with proper arrangement followed by 'coma'.

C) Source: Sources of rubrics are different Homoeopathic Materia Medica.

D) Construction of Rubric: It is the process of making the rubrics from various symptoms of MM.

   - While conversion of symptoms into rubrics following rules are adapted:
     - Convert the rubric with language of repertory used
     - Convert the language of the case to that of the repertory without mutilating its original meaning.

- Example:
1. Symptom – Throbbing type of pain in head relieved by pressure

   Rubric – Pain, sub rubric – pulsating, pressure amel. – Head section
2. Symptom – Patient has fear of death when alone

   Rubric – Fear, sub rubric – Death, sub-sub rubric alone when – Mind section

E) **Arrangement of rubrics:** Rubrics are arranged alphabetically under each and every section in different repertories.

   Example: Skin Section – Adherent, Anesthesia, Bedsore, Biting, Callous, Cancer

F) **Classification of rubrics:**
   1. General Rubric
   2. Particular Rubric

1) **General Rubrics** – Is the subheadings under different chapters (i.e. Main headings) covers larger no. of remedies. General rubrics are usually not modified by any sub rubric like side, time, character, extension etc.

   Ex – Pain, in Head – Having more than 500 remedies

   Such type of rubrics usually contains a larger no. of medicines. So as they are remedial common symptoms they have secondary importance in repertorial totality. But Kent writes while repertorization first work out general rubric followed by particular rubric to avoid missing similimum.

2) **Particular Rubrics** – These are nothing but sub-rubrics that is the result of modifications of rubrics either by site, time, modalities, extension, location, character of sensation and many other factors.

   Ex – Pain, Forehead, Amel Pressure – Carry limited no. of remedies deducted from General rubrics.

   Such rubric gives smaller number of remedies so useful for proper selection of remedy.

3) **SUB RUBRIC**
   - Sub Rubric is further Characterization, classification or Modification of rubric on the basis of certain conditions.

     Ex. Side, Time, Modalities, Extensions, Sensations, Locations, Adaptability, alternates with, Causation, Sensation as if, various types, Unexpected deviation etc.

     Example of sub rubric – From Kent's Repertory – Eye section

Following sub Rubrics modifies Rubric pain
   - Side – Right side, left side
   - Time – Daytime, Morning, Forenoon, Noon etc.
   - Modalities – arranged alphabetically air cold agg to Yawning
   - Extension – e.g. eye, pain, extending to frontal sinus
   - Sensation – e.g. eye, pain, aching, biting, boring, cutting, drawing etc
   - Location – e.g. Under conjunctiva, back, behind lids, canthi in, eyelids, eye brows etc.

- <u>Adaptability</u> – e.g. Pain in eye while reading
- <u>Alternates with</u> – e.g. Pain in eye alternates with the pain in the abdomen
- <u>Causation</u> – e.g. Pains in eye on reading and writing
- <u>Sensation as if</u> – e.g. Burning pain as if in sand
- <u>Various types</u> – e.g. discharges, milky white

4) SYMPTOM VS RUBRIC

	SYMPTOM	RUBRIC
Definition	External manifestation of internal derangement of vital force	Repertorial language in which a big sentence is expressed by few words with proper arrangement followed by 'coma'.
Word	Greek word "Symptoma"	Latin word "Rubrica"
Meaning	Which means any change	Which means heading or guiding rule
Types	General, particular, subjective objective etc.	General rubric, sub rubrics or sub divisions i.e. further modifications.
Source	Patient, physician, provers, attendance, laboratory investigation	Symptoms from different HMM that are converted into rubric
Utility in repertory	Has to be converted into rubric and then used for repertorization	As it is the language of the repertory used directly for repertorization
Gradation	Are graded in patient and in MM by definite principles	Rubrics are not graded but the grade of a symptom evaluates the importance of rubric for selection.
Analysis	Analyzed by different authorities and different ways	Rubrics are not analyzed
Character	Are incomplete	Are complete
Source	Patient, physician, provers, attendance,laboratory investigation	Symptoms from different HMM that are converted into rubric
Utility in repertory	Has to be converted into rubric and then used for repertorization	As it is the language of the repertory used directly for repertorization
Gradation	Are graded in patient and in MM by definite principles	Rubrics are not graded but the grade of a symptom evaluates the importance of rubric for selection.

5) CROSS REFERENCE

- Word meaning: Cross-reference means reference to another passage in the same book.
- Cross-reference is a useful way of making it easier to get through the repertory
- Definition: These are rubrics used instead of others that bear the same meaning when correctly interpreted (means substitute of one –With or without remedies)
- Types of Cross Reference

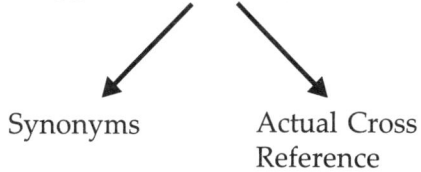

Synonyms   Actual Cross
                  Reference

e.g. In Kent's Repertory – (see rubric) this is for two purposes

- Synonyms – rubrics like abandoned (see forsaken)
- Cross reference – Rubrics like Absent – Minded (see forgetful)
- No list of medicines after the rubric indicates synonyms (Blind rubric) and list of medicines after the (see Rubric) means Cross-reference.
- These rubrics are having apparently same meaning but when carefully interpreted their lies some difference in the inner meaning. Remedies and sub rubrics are added to the most appropriate rubric.

  e.g. Absent –Minded (see forgetfulness)
- To use exact rubric one must know the inner meaning of each rubrics

  e.g. Hurry – does every thing hurriedly, i.e. work, eating etc.

  Impatience – cannot wait for any thing.

- Again one must ask to oneself that why there are cross references in repertory, the only reason is at the time of proving different prover expressed their feelings in their own words.

  e.g. in case of Thuja, prover first explained feeling of brittleness and the same feeling is expressed by another prover that as if he is made of glass.

- Cross references used in various repertories:
  - Kent's repertory – Dr. Kent has mentioned cross-references against rubrics in bracket wherever they are required.
  - Dr. Boger's Repertory – Dr. Boger has mentioned them at the end of chapters at one place.
  - Knerr's Repertory – Dr. Knerr has mentioned them with the sign of hand direct to the related symptoms, disease conditions.

  e.g. Abhorrence Aversion

- Advantages of Cross-references:
  - It helps to differentiate similar Rubrics.
  - It helps to locate the appropriate Rubrics.
  - It helps to compare drugs mentioned at both places.
  - Cross-reference helps to interpret the meaning of characteristic symptoms and convert them in to the appropriate rubric without any confusion.
  - Used to make new addition if any one wants to work on Repertory

6) REPERTORIAL TOTALITY (REPERTORIAL SYNDROME)

Before we go for the Repertorial concept i.e. Repertorization we need to elicit totality from various sources which are listed in aphorisms of Organon. Repertorial totality is a logical related group of signs and symptoms where three major concepts of totality and philosophy is considered.

Definition: It is the rearrangement of totality according to repertory used and method used for repertorization (whether Kent's Boenninghausen's Boger's etc.)

● This is also called as Repertorial Syndrome which is used to designate those symptoms, rubrics and their aggregates which are utilized for the purpose of repertorisation.

● The repertorial syndrome/totality varies according to the logic applied, the philosophical background and method selected as required by the case, i.e. from the three major schools.

● The symptoms or Rubrics selected for the repertorial syndrome form a hierarchy of importance of symptoms according to the philosophical background, what remains after deducting the repertorial totality from the conceptual image constitutes the potential difference.

● Conceptual image-Repertorial totality= Potential difference field

7) POTENTIAL DIFFERENCE

As totality changes from patient to patient, potential difference is also changing.

Potential difference is that symptomatology which remains after deducting repertorial totality from conceptual image.

Potential difference is considered for prescription but not for actual mathematical calculations.

It is a part of patients totality or remedies totality. Potential difference helps in differentiating group of remedies that comes after repertorisation and guides for individualizing the case.

e.g:

- Miasm
- Thermal status
- Diagnosis of the disease
- Acute & chronic phase of disease
- Physical Constitution
- Temperament
- Diathesis
- Side affinity
- Pathological generals

8) HUNTING OF RUBRICS

Definition: It is a method or process of searching out the required rubrics from the particular sections and locates the same in the repertory to study it in detail in relation to indicated remedies with their different grades.

● So for proper hunting of required rubric from any of the repertory one should know in detail:

- Plan and construction of the particular repertory.
- Philosophy and adaptability
- Scopes and limitations of various repertories
- Different typography used to grade the remedies and their abbreviations.

● To locate the proper rubric from mind section of any repertory requires knowing:

- Exact dictionary meaning of that rubric.
- Differentiating points of similar rubrics.
- Different cross-references.
- There are different techniques of hunting or rubrics:
  1. Scientific technique
  2. Direct technique

Scientific Technique

- It is an ideal technique where rubrics are searched by following systemic plan i.e.

  SECTION → SUB-SECTION (HEADING) → RUBRIC → SUB-RUBRIC

- Students and neophyte commonly use this technique. As compared to the other technique is time consuming but by following this, one will perfect in using the repertory.

Direct Technique

- In many of the repertories at last there is a word index, which helps to note the page number of the required rubric and open the referred page. This technique is less time consuming and used by busy practitioners who are expert in using the repertories, but not allowed for students in examination.

9) SYNTHESIS OF RUBRICS

Many times while working for the case with one of the repertory this happens that each and every required rubric is not found in that repertory but some other similar rubrics are observed. In this case if those similar rubrics are combined together one many get required rubric according to totality. This concept of combining different rubrics into one is called synthesis of rubrics.

So while repertorisation in such cases one can either consider all remedies from both rubrics or another option is consideration of only common remedies and others are eliminated.

10) GRADATION OF REMEDY

Gradation of remedy is qualitative value of remedy in provers as well as in patient.

The principle of gradation of remedies depends upon appearance of that symptom in the remedy during proving, reproving and clinical verification.

The credit of evaluating or grading or remedies goes to Dr. Boenninghausen, which he had used in his first Repertory i.e. 'Repertory of Antipsoric remedies'. He used five variations in type that indicated the individual evaluation of each remedy to the given symptom or rubrics. In different Repertories remedies are graded in different grades by using different typography:

Gradations of Medicines

Method	First grade	Second Grade	Third Grade
Recording of drug proving	Symptoms appear in every prover	Symptoms appear in few of the provers	Symptoms appear now and then in a proving
Confirmation reproving	Confirmed	Confirmed	Not yet Confirmed by reproving
Verification upon the sick	Verified clinically upon the sick	Occasionally Verified clinically upon the sick	Verified by having cured sick folks

Grade	BBCR/BTPB	Synthetic	Kent	Synoptic	PHATAK	Boericke
First	CAPITAL	CAPITAL	**Bold**	CAPITAL	CAPITAL	*Italics*
Second	**Bold**	CAPITAL	*Italics*	*Italics*	*Italics*	Roman
Third	*Italics*	**Bold**	Roman	Roman	Roman	
Fourth	Roman	Roman				
Fifth	(Roman)					

11) REPERTORIAL ANALYSIS

- **Definition**: Repertory analysis is conversion of patient's symptoms into repertorial language without changing its meaning.

- Repertory analysis differs with the construction and plan of repertory.

- Patient's symptoms can be converted into section, Rubric/Heading, Sub-rubric/sub-heading accordingly.

- e.g. Patient says I want to die because of pains.

- **Repertory Analysis:**

Repertory	Section	Rubric	Sub-rubric	Page No	Repertory
Kent	Mind	Suicidal, Dispo-sition	Pains from	85	Kent

12) REPERTORIAL RESULT ANALYSIS

After repertorisation and totalization of marks as per given marks from respective repertory, before prescribing any remedy from obtained group of remedies one must go for qualitative matching of each remedy out of group with that of evaluated symptoms of the patient.

For example, if after repertorial result one find that 3-4 remedies are running closely and carries almost equal marks and also covers equal number of symptoms out of considered totality, then in such case while prescribing one must try to match remedy qualitatively which means he must analyze each remedy separately in relation to marks obtained and for what symptoms it is obtained.

In homoeopathic practice qualitatively forming of totality plays important role that even while collecting symptoms from patient recording of grades of that symptom is required, because it should not happen that out of result of repertorisation one remedy has equal marks but that remedy covers third grade symptoms for higher marks and is running up with other remedies.

13) GENERALIZATION

Generalization is an aspect of the process of identification and applies forming general notions or formation of general concepts from particulars.

The concept is based on the principle, which is true to the part, is true to the whole.

Dictionary meaning of the generalization is to draw a general conclusion, speaks in general terms.

- Word meaning of General is - overall, not related to one, not specific.
- Generalize is a principle, theory with general application. So generalization is to form general principle or conclusion from detailed facts, experience etc. or the act of process of generalizing.

  So generalization is an act or a method to come at generals from specifics or particulars.
- Example - a person complaining of throbbing type of pain in eye. He also complaining of undefined pain in head. Here application or eye pain to head is generalization of sensations.
- According to Dr. Boenninghausen to get complete symptom generalization of modalities as well as sensation is possible.

14) PARTICULARIZATION
- Particularization is reverse process of generalization. Which is true to the part is true to the specific part.
- Word meaning of particular is relating to one person or thing and no others. So particular is specific to part.
- In homoeopathy these terms (Generalization & particularization) are referred to Dr. Boenninghausen, Dr. Kent's Repertory and Boger's work.
- The other work on BTPB i.e. BBCR is based on particularization.
- Kent's Repertory is based on generalization.
- With the concept of particularization Dr. Kent published his repertory and controversy started which tempted Dr. Boger to work on BTPB and he also followed concept of particularization by giving particular sensations and modalities separately.

- Dr. Kent says, throbbing type of pain in head is of head alone, similarly Headache ameliorates in open air is may not be sensation and modalities of the other part.

REPERTORISATION
- **Definition:** Repertorisation is an artistic and scientific method of individualization or generalization of patient in which the process is done by mathematical calculations of totality and their medicines with proper grades from the repertory.
- After repertory analysis according to method used and repertory used one should give the marks to the indicated remedies for respective rubrics then the total number of matched symptoms and the total marks of the medicines are calculated mathematically to get the group of remedies on the basis of maximum obtained marks and maximum covered symptoms. Lastly final selection is based on the knowledge of Materia Medica.

CROSS REPERTORIZATION
- There are several repertories, among them homoeopathic physicians in their practice generally use BTPB, BBCR and KRHMM.
- Other repertories have a limited use and they are mostly used for reference purposes.
- However, with the advent of many recent repertories like homoeopathic medical repertory, synthetic repertory and synthesis, the practitioners has a choice **and advantage of selecting any useful repertory for the case.**

- Selection of repertory for repertorization mainly depends on the type of the case and physician's acquaintance with the particular repertory.
- In day-to-day practice, a physician generally limits himself to one repertory while working out a case.
- The term cross repertorization is used when more than one repertory is consulted either to help the selection of similimum or to confirm the result obtained from the use of one repertory.
- A case can be repertorized by any repertory provided the case has a wide dimension, so that totality can be created from any angle – Kent, Boenninghausen and Boger.
- All such cases may be suitable for cross repertorization.
- Any case, which has various rubrics that are not found in one repertory, need reference of more than one repertory – in such cases too cross repertorization is required.
- The purpose of cross repertorization is to highlight the oneness of all repertories with regard to their objective, that is, to find out the similimum.
- Another purpose of cross repertorization is to select well represented rubric from any of the repertories.

Methods of Cross Repertorization

1. **Using one totality**
   - A case is selected for repertorization through a repertory and accordingly a totality is erected.
   - The same totality can be used for referring other repertories.

2. **Rearranging the totality**
   - In this method, the totality is rearranged according to the philosophy of different repertories.
   - Thus after taking the case, the evaluated symptoms are arranged logically which can be reconstructed according to different repertories.

3. **Integrated approach**
   - Under this method, one totality is erected in the first instance for repertorization.
   - Then rubrics should be referred to in all repertories and a note made regarding the availability of the rubrics.
   - The next step is to find out those repertories wherein these rubrics are represented well.
   - This is the most important approach, which helps to derive the maximum benefit from all existing repertories.
   - The well represented rubrics, selected from various repertories, are used for repertorization.
   - This approach leaves minimum error in repertorization, especially in respect of omission of drugs

SELECTION OF A PROPER REPERTORY

- After the totality has been erected, the case becomes clear to the physician.
- He should look for one of the following points in the case:

1. General: Mentals/Physicals
2. Particulars:
   i. Location
   ii. Sensation
   iii. Modalities
   iv. Concomitants
   v. Pathological generals

- If a case were full of generals, Kent's repertory would be the best selection.

- If it has got pathological generals, Boger's repertory must be selected.

- If the case has got particulars, with L, S, M, C with a few mentals, BTPB is preferable; however, Boger's repertory can also be used

- Once the repertory has been selected, the next step is to rearrange the totality according to the repertory selected.

- Rearrangement of totality in terms of the repertory selected is called Repertorial totality. Thus a well arranged totality is worked out.

- What follows next is to convert the symptoms into rubrics which requires an acquaintance with the repertory.

- The symptoms obtained from the patient many not be found in the repertory in the same form; so the physician must know the construction and arrangement of each repertory.

ERECTING TOTALITY

- Totality is not the sum total of symptoms but it is a logical combination of the symptoms, which characterize the person as well as individualizes the problem.

- Thus, all the symptoms, which are classified and evaluated, do not form a working totality of the case.

- From classification and evaluation, the hierarchy of symptoms is known, but which among them should be used for getting a correspondence, is yet to be finalized.

- Thus a physician is required to understand the whole symptom and to select a few which can logically represent the whole picture.

- This logical arrangement must follow a definite principle.

- If the case has go more generals and a few particulars with rare modalities, it would follow a different arrangement than that of a case, which has vague modalities and striking concomitants, or a pathological general.

- Totality should be erected according to the facts collected in the case.

- There is no hard and fast rule to erect the totality in any fixed way.

The case alone decides the method to be followed.

SECTION III

Author: Lippe

Published: 1879

Lippe's Repertory is based on 'The Repertory to the Manual' published in Allentown in 1838 by Hering.

It includes information from the literature of Guernsey, Hering, Jahr, Adolph von Lippe, Bell and Boenninghausen.

1st edition – 1879 by Boericke and Tafel

1st Indian edition – 1933 bt Bhattacharya and Co.

5th edition – 1972 by B. Jain Publishers

Lippe's Repertory can be divided into three parts:

Part I – Preface

Part II – Repertory

Part III – List of remedies

PHILOSOPHICAL BACKGROUND

Lippe followed deductive logic that is from general to particular, which was later adopted by Kent.

GRADATION

1st grade: Italics

2nd grade: Roman

NUMBER OF REMEDIES: 301

PLAN AND CONSTRUCTION

The repertory is divided into 34 chapters – starting from Mind and disposition up to Generalities – Aggravations and Ameliorations.

Rubrics are arranged alphabetically.

FEATURES

1. The repertory is based on the concept of deductive logic.

2. The method of construction is not fixed. It varies from section to section.

3. The chapter of **Generalities** mainly consists of aggravations and ameliorations, which is similar to that of Therapeutic Pocket Book.

4. Some mental symptoms are misplaced and are included in Generalities.

5. Concomitant symptoms in relation to stool, urination, menses are included in Generalities as well as in respective sections.

6. Rubrics in relation to **food and drinks** are mentioned alphabetically. Kent grouped them into aversions and desires

7. Rubrics of **temperaments** are given alphabetically. Boger included them under the rubric Temperament.

8. There is a special note in the Preface, stating that all sections are to be compared with the section "Generalities".

10. **Time modalities** are arranged alphabetically. Kent includes them at the beginning in chronological order.

11. **Pain** sensations are arranged alphabetically by Lippe. Kent arranged them under the rubric Pain.

LIPPE'S INFLUENCE OVER KENT

A need was felt by Kent for a new and a more complete and useful repertory. Initially, Kent used Therapeutic Pocket Book but was soon dissatisfied with its philosophy and he started to go through the repertories published up to that time.

The first step in this direction was the Repertory to the more Characteristic Symptoms of our Materia Medica by Constantine Lippe. In this repertory modalities were given in detail. The concepts were broadened and put to maximum benefit In Kent's repertory.

He liked the plan and arrangement of Lippe's repertory.

Dr. Kent had a thorough knowledge of Materia Medica and he found that many medicines were lacking in Lippe's repertory. So he added notes to each symptom or rubric. This was interleaved many times. Hence Kent got into contact with Lippe, who wanted Kent to work along with Lee who was preparing a 3rd edition of Lippe's repertory. By this time Dr. Kent had prepared a repertory of urinary organs, chill, fever, sweat, etc.

Hence, it can be said that Lippe's work was the base for Kent's Repertory.

INTRODUCTION:

Dr.Kent was an eclectic practioner and was converted to homoeopathy when his wife suffered from insomnia and was treated by Dr. Phelan with Pulsatilla. He started studying Hahnemann's Organon.

During his time Boennighausen's and Lippe's repertory were commonly used in practice. He also studied Biegler's Diary, Minton's Diseases of Women and Jahrs repertory. He liked the form and character of Lippes repertory but was not satisfied with the rubrics and number of medicines used. As he studied Lippes repertory he wrote the observations in the margins and in between lines in Lippes repertory. So, to fill the lacunae he took the task of writing a repertory and talked to Dr.Lee of Philadelphia as Lippes abridged form of new repertory was with Lee. Lippe desired that Kent and Lee should work together but at that time , Dr. Kent had completed a repertory on urinary organs, chills, fever and sweat with other sections partially completed. Lee with the help of Dr.Kent compiled mind and head sections but it was not upto the expectations of Dr.Kent as it was based on Boennighausen's idea of generals and modalities were given at the end of the book. Later, Lee became blind and Dr.Kent revised and rearranged the book according to his own plan which chiefly followed **Lippes Handbook of Characteristics.** Dr. Kent started using it in his own practice. When asked by Dr. Beigler about the book Dr. Kent expressed difficulty in publishing it on account of huge cost involved in it. Then Dr.Biegler, Dr.Kimball and Thurston helped him to get enough subscribers and then it was published part by part.

1) Ist edition was published in 1897(1428 pages).

2) 2 nd edition between 1900 to 1901.

3) 3 rd edition in 1924 under assistance of F.E.Gladvin, J.S.Pugh, published by Dr. Ehrhrt and Karl.

4) 4 th edition in 1935 published with the help of Dr. Clara Kent, Dr.Gladvin and Dr.Pierre Schimdt.

5) 5 th edition came in 1945 published by Dr. Ehrhrt and Karl.

6) 6th edition came in 1957 published by Dr. Ehrhrt and Karl.

7) First Indian edition came out in 1961.

A revised version of Kent was published by Dr.Pierre Schmidt in 1974, who compiled this corrected version with the original work of Kent, but when it was ready for publication it was stolen , Dr. Diwan Harishcandra salvaged it in the multilated form it is called revised first edition or Final general repertory of Kent.

Sources of Kents Repertory:

a) Lippe's Repertory

b) Biegler's diary

c) Jahr's Repertory

d) Allen's Symptom Register

e) Allen's Great Encyclopaedia

f) Minton's Diseases of women

PHILOSOPHIC BACKGROUND

Kent's repertory is based on philosophy of Deductive logicie, from general to particular. He has given importance to general symptoms as according to him "Man prior to organs". He criticized the faulty method of giving importance to parts and over generalizing the symptoms. Kent used earlier material medicas and clinical observations but didn't took those drugs which were insufficiently confirmed.

It contains 648 medicines. Some studies says that it has 591 medicines, as per Dr.R.P.Patel the number of medicines were 657.

There are three typographies used in the repertory:

1) Bold Letter 3 marks   First Grade

2) Italics   2 marks   Second grade

3) Ordinary   1 mark   Third grade

First grade symptoms are recorded in majority of provers, confirmed and verified

Second grade symptoms are recorded in few provers and are occasionally verified

Third grade symptoms are very few provers and lack clinical confirmation .

PLAN AND CONSTRUCTION

In order to study this repertory it can be divided into three parts:

1) First part has

Use of the repertory: Dr.Kent

How to study the repertory:- Dr.Kent

Repertorisation by Dr. Margaret Tyler and Dr.John Weir

Hot and Cold remedies by Dr. Gibson

Cases demonstration by Dr.M.L Tyler and Dr.John Weir

2) Second part : Repertory proper

Preface by Dr.Kent

Contents of various sections (37)

List of remedies with abbreviations

Repertory

Word index

3) Third part:

Sides of body and drug affinities from Boennighausens lesser writing

Relationship of remedies with duration of action by Gibson Miller

The plan and construction of chapters also follows generals to particulars.1st chapter is Mind and last Chapter is Generalities. There are total 33 chapters in Kent out of which the chapter on urinary organs is having 5 subdivisions(32+5=37).So, one can say that there are 37 chapters in Kents repertory excluding word index. It has 1434 pages.

Systematic arrangement of chapters

• Central Nervous System – (Mind, Vertigo, Head)

• Special Senses With Its Functions(Eye, Vision, Ear, Hearing, Nose)

• Face

• Gastrointestinal System (Mouth, Teeth, Throat, Stomach, Abdomen, Rectum, Stool)

• External Throat Comes After Throat

• Genitourinary System (Bladder, Kidneys, Prostate, Urethra, Urine, Genitalia Male, Genitalia Female)

• Respiratory System (Larynx & Trachea, Respiration, Cough, Expectoration, Chest)

• Cardiovascular System (Chest)

- Locomotor System (Back, Extremities)
- Sleep
- Stages Of Fever (Chill, Fever, Perspiration)
- Skin
- Generalities

In the arrangement of chapters structures are followed by functions

- Eye, vision
- Ear, hearing
- Exception – respiration, chest

ARRANGEMENT OF RUBRICS

Rubrics

Rubrics are arranged in alphabetical order.

Rubrics are represented in bold roman letters.

Rubrics are arranged from generals to particulars i.e. it starts with a general rubric followed by particular rubrics with exceptions.

Many rubrics start with particular rubrics – e.g. Nose, Discharge, right.

Rubrics & medicines are separated by a colon.

Medicines are separated by a semicolon.

Medicines are given in alphabetical order with gradations.

In rubrics medicines are given as abbreviations , index of which is given in the beginning of repertory.

Sub rubrics

Sub rubrics are represented with ordinary roman letters with locations as exception which is given as a separate heading.

Subrubrics are arranged under the rubric with indentation to the right.

Subsubrubrics are arranged under the subrubrics with indentation to the right.

Subrubrics are arranged in STME pattern ie side, time, modalities, extension with many exceptions.

STME pattern is inappropriate to represent the arrangement of subrubrics in kents repertory.

STMEL is a better pattern to represent the arrangement of subrubrics , ie side ,time , modalities, extension, locations.

Generally all sub rubrics are in STMEL pattern except at some places.

In a set of rubrics, time is given after modalities, i.e. , MT pattern instead of TM

TIME rubrics.

Side
- Side is not given in alphabetical order
- Right is given first then left

Time

Time is arranged under rubrics in the order of sunrise to sunset followed by night with the exception of daytime

- Day time – dawn – dusk (6am – 6pm)
- Morning – (6 am — 8 am) – (9 am — 11 am)
- Forenoon – (8am — 11 am) – 12pm
- Noon — 12 pm – 1 pm
- Afternoon – 1pm – (5pm – 6 pm)
- Evening – (6pm – 9pm), twilight
- Night – 9 pm – 6 am, it includes sub rubrics like midnight before, midnight, midnight after.

In some chapters midnight is given as a separate rubric. E.g – Chill.

Defects of time arrangement
- Clock timings overlap at many places
- Difficult to find out a particular time
- Rubrics & subrubrics over laps
- Does not follow arrangement — STME

Modalities
Modalities are arranged in alphabetic order

It includes aggravations, ameliorations, concomitants, alternations, causations, accompaniments.

Locations
Locations are not directly represented in Kent's repertory.

Locations are represented under sensations or modalities (ie under rubrics) with some exceptions.

Locations are given directly at some places

Eg. Liver, Spleen, pancreas.

Locations are represented under rubrics after the completion of STME pattern of general rubric & given in bold roman letters as a separate section but as a part of the rubric under which STME pattern is followed.

Locations are also represented at the end of the general rubric as normal subrubrics ie after extension.

Locations are arranged under the rubric in anatomical order& in alphabetical order.

Anatomical order – Extremities

Alphabetical order – Head, Throat, Abdomen, Genitalia male.

In chest locations are given in alphabetical order except for the heart which is given at the end of locations.

Head – Brain, Occiput, Sides, Temples, Vertex, Forehead, Hair.

Eye – Margins, Conjunctiva, Canthi, Lids, Lachrymal Glands, Eye Brows, Iris, Lachrymal Canal, Lachrymal Sac, Meibomian Glands, Retina, Optic Nerve,

Ear – Concha, Eustachian Tube, Antitragus, Lobule, Tragus.

Nose – Root, Posterior Nares, Septum, Tip, Wings.

Face – Cheek, Chin, Infra Orbital, Lips, Jaw, Articulation, Mental Foramen, Parotid Gland, Submaxillary Gland, Zygoma, Sub Lingual Gland.

Mouth – Gums, Palate, Tongue, Inside Of Lips.

Teeth – Incisors, Canines, Molars, Upper Teeth, Lower Teeth, Bicuspid.

Throat – Oesophagus, Oshyoids, Tonsils, Pharynx, Uvula, Fauces.

External Throat – Carotids, Thyroid Gland, Jugular, Cervical Glands.

Stomach – Stomach

Abdomen – Mesentrics, Region Of Hip, Caecal Region, Liver, Spleen, Inguinal Region, Sides Of Abdomen, Lower Abdomen, Muscles Of Abdomen, Hypochondrium, Hypogastrium, Umbilicus, Ileocaecal Region.

Rectum – Perineum, Between Nates, Anus

Bladder – Neck Of Bladder, Region Of Blader, Sphincter.

Kidneys – Ureter, Region Of Kidneys

Prostate Gland – Prostate, Region Of Prostate.

Urethra – Anterior Part Of Urethra, Fossa Navicularis, Meatus, Glandular Portion Of Urethra.

Genitalia Male – Penis, Scrotum, Testes, Spermatic Cord, Prepuce, Glans Penis, Fraenum, Root Of Penis.

Genitalia Female – Ovaries, Vagina, Uterus, Cervix.

Larynx & Trachea – Larynx, Trachea, Throat Pit, Epiglottis.

Chest – Axillae, Lungs, Mammae, Region Of Heart, Heart, Nipples, Sternum, Clavicles, Lowerpart Of Chest, Middle Of Chest, Sides Of Chest, Upper Part Of Chest, Pleura, Diaphragm, Endocardium, Pericardium, Pectoral Muscles.

Back – Cervical Region, Dorsal Region, Lumbar Region, Sacral Region, Spine, Scapular Region, Between Shoulders, Sacrum, Coccyx, Scapulae, Ilium, Iliac Crest, Lumbo Sacral Region, Sacro Iliac Junction.

Extremities – Psoas, Nates, Lower Limbs, Upper Limbs,Shoulder Joint, Humerus, Upper Arm, Elbow, Fore Arm, Hand, Metacarpal Bone, Wrist, Fingers, Thumb, Finger Joints, Hip, Femur, Thigh, Knee, Tibia, Fibula, Leg, Ankle Joint, Foot, Heel, Toes, Toe Nails, Soles.

Pain

Pain starts as in general followed by STME pattern , types of pain in alphabetical order with subrubrics in STME pattern -Eye, ear, nose, throat, kidneys, extremities.

In Head, chest, male genitalia pain is not followed by sides but sides are given under locations only.

In abdomen, face pain starts with particular types – aching not with pain in general.

In mouth, penis pain in general have no subrubrics & immediately followed by locations with subrubrics & with particular type of pains.

In teeth pain starts with locations followed by STME pattern.Under some locations side is given.

In generalities pain starts with the appearance of pain followed by locations followed by type of pains in alphabetical order.

Cross references

Cross references are given soon after the rubic or subrubric in brackets.

Cross references contains medicines in both or all rubrics. Cross references means rubrics with similar meaning & used in different context.

SCOPES OF KENTS REPERTORY

1) It is based on philosophy of generals to particulars and rubrics are also arranged like this which makes it easy to use.

2) It is having 648 medicines which is more than Therapeutic pocket book and Boger's repertory.

3) It has three gradations which makes it more practical for use.

4) Generalities section is large and elaborate and contain many subrubrics which are useful.

5) Rubrics and subrubrics are arranged alphabetically making the search easier.

6) Mind section contains many rubrics and sub rubrics and also contains qualified symptoms which are helpful in repertorising.

7) Cross references are given in paranthesis immediately after rubric.

8) It contains rubrics related to parts as well as to generals so there is no need to refer another repertory.

LIMITATIONS OF KENTS REPERTORY

1) At some places medicines seen under sub rubrics are not seen at main rubrics

   E.g: Delusion general rubric: Dros is not seen

   But in subrubrics

   Delusion , persecuted he is- Dros

   Delusion , longer things seem- Dros

2) He criticized Boennighausen's Therapeutic Pocket Book for listing medicines under parts but he himself could not avoid use of them e.g.: Pancreas, spleen, Affections of Heart

3) His repertory is having many clinical rubrics which do not justify his philosophy , e.g.: Pneumonia, oedema, anaemia.etc.

4) There are many similar rubrics which confuses the beginner e.g.: Chargin, sadness.

5) Though kent used nosodes it is not represented well in the repertory

6) There is over generalization in mind chapter and over particularization in extremities chapter.

7) Many rubrics suffer from omission of drugs e.g.: Faintness, menses during- Cyclamen

8) Many rubrics have single medicines which cannot be used for repertorisation, e.g.: Consolation, amel- Puls is only mentioned

9) Kent has given importance to thermal conditions but there is not a single rubric which can be referred to in this aspect.

10) Some of the general modalities, which should be mentioned in generalities, also appear in parts.

    E.g: Wetting feet agg - Extremities

    Wet feet generalities

Relative significance of Kent repertory

Biggest Chapter in Kent's Repertory:- Extremities (281 pages).

Smallest Chapter- Hearing (2 Pages)

Largest rubric in mind Chapter- Delusion .

The drugs are of three Gradings.

1. Well proved, clinically verified drugs - Represented in Bold, those symptoms produced by majority of   provers and frequently verified.

2. Occasionally proved drugs - Represented in italics produced by few provers and occasionally verifed

3. Only in small group of provers - Represented in roman

The grading of the drugs will help in easy and fast repertorisation without compromising results.

The grading of remedies are done as mentioned above and the source for it is :

1) Drug-Proving

2) Toxicological evidence

3) Clinical experience

Name of the book: Boenninghausen's therapeutic pocket book for Homoeopathic Physicians to used at Bedside and in the study of Homoeopathic Materia Medica

Introduction : Dr. H .A. Roberts & Dr. Annie C Wilson.

Publisher : B. Jain Publishers Pvt. Ltd , New Delhi.

Year of Publishing: 1935

Reprint Edition : 1994

First Edition : 1846

Total pages : 503

INTRODUCTION

Contents:

Part I

Preface

Life History of Boenninghausen

Part II

Repertory Proper

Index

Repertory Uses

The art of physician in taking the case

The philosophic Background

Construction of the Repertory

Introduction to different Chapters

- Mind and intellect

- Parts of the Body and Organs

- Sensations and complaints

- Sleep and Dreams

- Fever

- Alterations of State of Health

- Relationships of Remedies

Limitations of Repertory

Use of the Analysis

Preface to the New American Edition

Boenninghausen's Original Preface

Part. I

Preface by Dr. T.F. Allen

In the preface Dr. T.F. Allen says that his aim is to demonstrate the sound philosophy and practical application of this work to such state as the physician meets in everyday practice. He admits that the book is not perfect but the principles upon which it is based are sound and will allow further expansion without distorting the basic principles.

Life History of Boenninghausen He was born in Netherlands. There is a controversy about the birth year of Boenninghausen, according to Lippe it is 1777. But in the beginning of the chapter the year given is 1785.

H.A. Roberts and Annie. C. Wilson gives a brief sketch of Boenninghausen's life and they show how a lawyer turned to an expert Homoeopath. It was Dr. Weihe who influenced Boenninghausen by rescuing him from the purulent tuberculosis with the help of Pulsatilla.

Authors give works of Boenninghausen in their order of appearance. They are:

1. The cure of cholera and its preventives 1831.

2. Repertory of Antipsoric Medicines 1832.

3. Summary View of the Chief Sphere of Operation of the Antipsoric Remedies and of their characteristic Peculiarities, as an appendix to their Repertory 1833.

4. An attempt at a Homoeopahtic Therapy of Intermittent fever 1833.

5. Contributions to a Knowledge of the Peculiarities of Homoeopahtic Remedies1833.

6. Homoeopahtic Diet and a Complete Image of a Disease 1833.

7. Homoeopathy a Manual for the Non-Medical Public1834.

8. Repertory of Medicines which are not Antipsoric 1835.

9. Attempt at showing the Relative Kinship of Homoeopahtic Medicines 1836.

10. Therapeutic manual for Homoeopahtic Physicians, for use at the sick bed and in the study of the Materia Medica Pura 1846.

11. Brief Instructions for Non- Physicians as to the Prevention and Cure of Cholera 1849.

12. The two sides of Human body and Relationships. Homoeopahtic studies 1853.

13. The Homoeopahtic domestic Physician in Brief Therapeutic Diagnosis. An attempt 1853.

14. The Homoeopahtic treatment of Whooping Cough in its Various Forms 1860.

15. The Aphorisms of Hippocrates with Notes by a Homoeopath 1863.

16. Attempt at a Homoeopathic Therapy of Intermittent and Other Fevers, especially for would- be Homoeopaths 1864.

Uses of repertory

Definition: Repertory is an index of symptoms arranged systematically. The system of arrangement may be founded upon certain definite guiding principles, or it may be alphabetical or schematic.

Uses:

1. To serve as a reference or a guide in looking up a particular symptom that may indicate the similimum or that may make necessary distinction between two or more similar remedies in a given case.

2. For careful study of all the symptoms that may appear in a c/c case. A repertory is not meant for those cases in which there is clear indication for the similimum.

The Value of Repertory

Depends upon several elements:

1. The art of physician in taking the case.

2. Knowledge of the Repertory one attempt to use; as regards
   a) Its philosophic background
   b) Its construction
   c) Its limitations
   d) Its adaptability

3. Intelligent use of the resulting analysis.

The art of physician in taking the case

Boenninghausen observed that, even with best possible case taking the case record is often left incomplete, one of the elements of symptom -ie., Location, sensation, modality or concomitant may be missing. He collected all such symptoms as they appeared in the cases; which came to him for treatment. Every case was examined symptomatically with the purpose to make every symptom as complete in itself as possible. Later he learned that, symptoms which existed in an incomplete state in some part could be completed by observing the conditions of other parts of the case.

This is called the doctrine of Analogy. He also discovered that, condition of aggravation or amelioration are not confined to a particular symptom, but they are like the red thread in the cordage of the British Navy, are applicable to all symptoms of the case. So he raised them (i.e. Particulars) to the level of Generals – It is called the doctrine of grand generalisation. It is the patient who is sick, not his head, nor his eyes nor his heart. Every symptom that refers to a part may be predicated of the whole man.The symptoms of disease are offen broken up and scattered through different parts of a patient. These scattered parts must be found and brought together in harmonious relation according to a typical form. This complete picture of the disease will give the totality.

Boenninghausen has designed his pocket book in such a way that, it would enable the physician to bring the symptoms together and complete one part by another.

- Primary symptoms: Symptoms which seemed to have a direct bearing on the complaint.

- Secondary symptoms : They belong to the class of concomitants.

- Typical symptom : Common symptom or disease symptoms

- Atypical symptoms :Symptoms, which belong to the individual. They are theconcomitants of disease symptoms.

PHILOSOPHIC BACKGROUND

It was with the encouragement of Hahnemann, that Boenninghausen developed his first repertory: Repertory of Antipsorics (1832). In 1835 he published Repertory of medicines which are not Antipsoric, in 1836 Attempt at showing the relative kinship of Homeopathic medicines and in 1846 he published, Therapeutic manual for Homoeopahtic physicians.

BTP is a combination of all these four books. The original book was written in German, it was first translated by one most eminent Homoeopathic physician. This translation was not practical. Later Alien made an edition; which suffered from faulty translation. Lastly in 1935 this Book was edited by Dr. H.A. Robert and Annie C. Wilson. Boenninghausen emphasized more on completing the symptom with all their components; i.e.

Location

Which includes parts, organs, tissues, systems as well as directions and extensions.

Sensation

Kind of pain, suffering and complaints, and also functional or organic changes characterising the morbid process.

Modality

This includes conditions of aggravation or ameliorations. Factors which cause, excite, increase or decrease or modify a symptom are included in the modality.

Concomitant

Symptoms appear and disappear with the main complaints; but they does not have any pathological relationship with the main complaints.

BTPB is based upon the following fundamental concepts:

1. Doctrine of analogy and doctrine of grand generalisation.

2. Doctrine of concomitant.

3. Evaluation of Remedies.

4. Concordances.

1. Doctrine of analogy/doctrine of grand generalization.

To make a symptom complete, the local modalities and sensations pertaining to one part should be applicable to other parts; in case modalities and sensations are not experienced by the patient or unnoticed by the Physician. Thus he raised local symptoms to a general level which could be used for the whole person. This principle is called doctrine ofAnalogy/doctrine of Grand Generalisation, He considered sickness as expression of the whole man, and not of the part. Sickness is expressed through different parts of the person. Thus all those modalities which are noticed in one part, but missing in any other part should be taken as an expression of the whole person.

2. Doctrine of concomitant

Boenninghausen, identified in each case a group of symptoms along with the main complaint; such symptoms were generally overlooked by the patient, and un noticed by the physician. He emphasized that, in all cases such a group of symptoms does exist, and they are missed, because of inadequate observation. They appear to be unrelated to the main complaint; but are quite crucial in individualizing the case as well as the remedy.

3. Evaluation of remedies

Boenninghausen was the first to grade the remedies. He noticed that there is difference in the frequency and intensity in the appearance of symptoms in provers. He graded the remedies into 5 grades – or marks.

He used different typography to represent these different grades of remedies.

A. CAPITAL to represent

1st Grade (5 marks)

Proved (Recorded)

Reproved (confirmed)

Clinically verified.

B. Bold to represent

2nd Grade (4 marks) Proved (less than the1st grade)

Reproved

(Confirmed) occasionally Verified.

C. Italics to represent
IIIrd Grade (3 marks)
Now and then a prover brings out symptom,
Not confirmed.
But verified
Clinically verified.

D. Roman to represent
IVth Grade (2 marks)
Only clinically verified

E. (Roman) in parenthesis represents
Vth Grade
One mark
Not confirmed
Not verified
Doubtful remedies.
But proved.

4. Concordances

He discusses the relationship of remedies; under headings – mind,locality, sensation, glands, bones skin, sleep and dreams, blood, circulation, fever, aggravation, other remedies, antidotes and inimical. Other remedies covers all the symptoms, which do not full into such regulars groups.

Plan and construction

The whole book can be divided into 3 components of a symptom – Location, sensation, and modalities. However concomitants are found scattered. Plan of Alien's modified edition:

I   Mind and Intellect

II   PARTS OF THE BODY

III. Sensations and Complaints
   - Sensations - In general
   - Sensations - Glands
   - Sensations - Bones
   - Sensations - Skin

IV   Sleep and Dreams

V   Fever

VI. Modalities

VII Relationship of remedies.

Part II

Introduction to different Chapters

1. Mind and Intellect

Mind Chapter contains 18 rubrics and Intellect Chapter contains 17 rubrics. In order to clarify the use of the book he simplified the number of rubrics as far as possible. Boenninghausen based his work on the concept of the whole man, placing the balance of the emphasis on the value of concomitants and the modalities. It was not his intention to reflect the whole man through his mental reactions, as they may be difficult to get. Eventhough this chapter contains only 35 rubrics the aggravation chapters include 17 rubrics related to emotional excitement or state.

The first rubric " Disposition generally affected" include medicines which affect the mind in general.

The rubric " Amativeness" which means inclined towards love and

" Mistrust" are not seen in kent's repertory.

Word meaning of some rubrics

Avarice = greedy, miserly

Boldness = daring, "Courageous" in Kent's repertory. But there is no medicine.

Fretfulness = peevishness, to irritated. Though this rubric is seen in Kent's repertory it contains no medicine.

Gentleness = Mildness, no medicine is given under " Gentleness" in Kent's repertory

Haughtiness = Pride

Activity = excitement

Befogged = confusion. The rubric " Befogged "is not found in Kent's repertory.

Comprehension difficult = Dullness

Ecstasy = exhilaration

Imaginations = fantastic illusions

Misplaced rubrics

Unconsciousness – this should have been given under sensations chapter.

Vertigo – there is no separate chapter. Since it is a sensation it should have bee given under "sensation" chapter.

Though he has given emphasis to the Concomitants in case taking, the concomitants of mental symptoms are given under a single rubric "Drugs which have concomitants of Mental Symptoms."

2. Parts of the body and organs

This section of the book follows in general the anatomical schema used by Hahnemann. T.F. Allen added many of the rubrics in the eye section. He also used an idea of combining Boenninghausen's

Repertory of the Sides of the Body with the original Pocket Book. This section on the parts of the body runs from page 24 to page 142, beginning with Chapter Internal Head and ending with Lower Extremities.

1. Internal Head:

The chapter begins with rubric- " Ineneral". Next different portions of head are given as rubrics - as

- Forehead
- Temples
- Sides of head
- Vertex
- Occiput

The chapter ends with the rubric – One sided in general.

There is no definite order of arrangement of the rubrics.

2. External Head:

Rubrics

- Hair
- Scalp
- Skull
- Beard
- Margins of hair

Are given in the chapter "External Head" Misplaced rubrics

a) Motion of Head

b) General sensations in External Head

c) Behind the Ears

The first two rubrics should have been given in the chapter "sensations" and the third one in the "ear" chapter.

The chapter "External Head" ends in the page number 29, in which the Chapter"

Internal Head" again begins. This contains only two rubrics – "Left side and Right side." The Chapter "External Head" is seen again with same rubrics in the page 30 where the second Chapter on "Internal Head" ends.

3. Eyes:

It contains rubrics like
- Aqueous humor
- Eye balls
- Choroid
- Conjunctiva
- Cornea
- Lachrymal apparatus
- Lens (Cataract)
- Optic nerve
- Retina
- White of eye (sclerotic)
- Brows
- Canthi
- Lids
- Orbits
- Sides - left and right

Misplaced rubrics:
- Adhesions in pupils
- Pupils Dilated
- Pupils Immovable
- Lachrymation
- Squinting
- Staring

They should have been given under the Chapter " Sensations"

4. Vision:

Here Boenninghausen is deviated from his original Philosophy. "Vision" which is a Sensation is given as a separate chapter among the parts of the body.

All the rubrics in this chapter and the Chapter as such can be considered as Misplaced.

Main rubrics in this Chapter include:
- Blindness
- Flickering
- Double
- Half vision
- Muscae Volitantes
- Dim
- Far-sighted
- Paralysis of Optic Nerve
- Photophobia
- Short –sighted

5. Ears:

This includes rubrics like;
- External
- Internal
- Middle ear (confounded with Internal)
- Eustachian Tube
- Lobules

Misplaced rubrics:

a) Parotid Glands- this might have been given under the Chapter Face

b) Discharges from Ears –

c) Ear-wax -

The last two rubrics might have been given under the Chapter Sensations according to the Philosophy of Boenninghausen.

6. Hearing :

It include rubrics like:
- Acute

- Hardness
- Loss of Hearing (from Paralysis of Auditory Nerve)
- Stopped Feeling ; etc

The Chapter along with its rubrics are out of place in the "Parts of the Body". They should have been given under the "Sensations".

7. Nose:

- External
- Internal
- Bones
- Root
- Septum
- Wings, etc are the main rubrics concerning the nose. But this Chapter contains many rubrics concerned with the sensations and complaints. They are
- Nose bleed
- Nasal catarrh
- Stopped Coryza
- Nasal Discharges
- Sneezing
- Ineffectual efforts to sneeze

The Chapter ends with Concomitants that are condensed into a single rubric – "Accompanying Symptoms of Nasal Discharges" and sides of nose" Left side and Right side"

8. Smell:

This include rubrics
- Sensitive
- Weak or Lost
- Illusions of Smell in General

The Chapter along with its rubrics should have been in Sensation Chapter.

9. Face:

The objective symptom that may be observed in the face is given first. Followed by locations of sensations.

The important rubrics include:
- Color - Bluish - Around Eyes
- Color - pale
- Circumscribed Redness of Cheeks
- Comedones
- Drawn
- Emaciation
- Expression Altered
- Eyes protruding
- Eyes- Sunken
- Freckles
- Open mouth
- Wrinkles – On forehead

The typography of Locations of sensations are given as a separate Chapter this may create confusion among the users. This include
- Forehead
- Temples
- Malar bones
- Cheek
- Upper Jaw
- Lower jaw
- Articulation of Jaws
- Lips
- Corners of lips
- Chin

And finally the Sides - Left and Right

10. Teeth:

It begins with "Toothache in General" Followed by different types of tooth namely,
- Incisors

- Eye teeth = Canine teeth
- Molars
- Gums (in Kent gums are given under Mouth Chapter)

Misplaced rubrics:

Hollow teeth = Caries of teeth
Teeth - Grinding

11. Mouth:

.Misplaced rubrics include (it should have been included under Sensations)

- Odor from Mouth
- Breath cold
- Breath hot
- Saliva diminished
- Saliva increased
- Tongue coated

The other rubrics include

Mouth in General

Tongue

Hard palate

Soft palate

12. Throat:

It include only the internal throat Tonsils are given under throat.

13. Mouth and fauces:

The Chapter on Mouth which ends on the page 64 again start on the page 65 as - Mouth and fauces in which the Sides ; Left and Right are given.

14. Hunger and Thirst:

This chapter should not have been given under the Heading of Parts of the Body. This might have been given as a separate Chapter or along with the Sensations.

The important rubrics include

Loss of appetite

Hunger

Thirst

Aversion and

Desires

15. Taste:

This include rubrics like

Altered in General

Acid

Bitter

Metallic

Nauseous

Salty

Sweetish

Lost

Taste being a special sensation; it along with its rubrics should be given in the Sensation Chapter.

16. Eructation's:

Belching

Hiccough

Uprisings

Waterbrash

Etc are given in this Chapter. The chapter as well as its rubrics is misplaced.

17. Nausea and Vomiting:

This include

Nausea in General

Qualmishness

Retching

Loathing

Vomiting and nature of vomiting

18. Internal Abdomen:

Stomach

Diaphragm

Hypochondria

Liver

Spleen

Epigastrium

Umbilical region

Loins

Groins (including Coecum, coecal region, ilio- coecal region, iliac region and Pourpart's Ligament)

Inguinal Rings

Sides

Are given in Internal Abdomen. In this the Loins are again given in the Extremities on Page 135.

Hernia is the only one Misplaced rubric.

19. External Abdomen:

Pit of stomach

Mons Veneris

Inguinal glands

Are given under External Abdomen

20. Abdomen :

The sides of Abdomen are mentioned in this separate Chapter which appears on the page number 81.

21 and 22. Hypochondria and Abdominal rings

These two chapters are mentioned as different chapters in the pages 82 and 83 respectively only to mention Left and Right sides.

23. Flatulence:

Flatulence in General

Borborygmi

Incarceration of Flatus

Are given in this Misplaced Chapter

24. Stool:

This chapter contains the following misplaced rubrics.

- Diarrhoea
- Constipation
- Worms
- Round worms
- Tape worms
- Thread worms
- Tenesmus
- Anus
- Haemorrhoids
- Rectum
- Perineum

This chapter also includes certain concomitant symptoms like

Troubles before stool

During stool

After stool

25. Urinary Organs:

Kidney

Bladder

Urethra

Are given in this chapter

Prostate is given in this chapter which is a misplaced rubric.

26. Urine:

Glycosuria can be taken for Diabetes Mellitus

Sediment in general can be used for urinary calculi.

27. Micturition:

Tenesmus of bladder

Dysuria

Involuntary

Retention of urine etc are some important misplaced rubrics.

Some concomitant rubrics are also given Troubles before Micturition

- During Micturition
- After Micturition

28. Sexual Organs:

The chapter starts with the rubric Sexual Organs in General, followed by Male Organs in General. It is followed by different parts of the Male genitalia-, Testicles Penis, Glans, Forskin, Scrotum and spermatic cord. The chapter also include rubrics for female Organs in General. Vagina, Uterus, Ovaries are given as separate rubrics.

Misplaced rubrics in this Chapter include: Labor- like Pains

Labor Pains Cease

After Pains

Desire Too Weak

-Too strong

Discharge of prostatic Fluid

Emissions

Erections

Impotency

Weak Sexual Power

The chapter ends with rubrics referring to the sides

Left and Right sides.

29. Menstruation

The chapter as well as the rubrics are out of place in this Main Chapter Parts of the body. The main rubrics include

Abortion

Menstruation Beginning, Delayed in Girls

- profuse
- scanty
- short
- suppressed

    Menses clotted

- Membranous

The concomitants of Menstruation are given at the end of the chapter

Before Menstruation

At Beginning of Menstruation

During Menstruation

After Menstruation

30. Leucorrhoea:

Various types of leucorrhoea and Accompanying Troubles of Leucorrhoea are given in this chapter.

31. Respiration:

It include important rubrics like

Arrested

Catching

Irregular

Oppressed

Rattling

Sighing

Suffocative Attacks

Concomitants of respiration are given in a single rubric

Accompanying Troubles of Respiration

32. Cough:

There is no separate chapter for Expectoration hence rubrics concerned with the Expectoration are given in this chapter. Chapter also include concomitant of cough which is given as last rubric – Troubles Associated with Cough.

33. Air-Passages:

It includes

Larynx &

Trachea

Some misplaced rubrics are found in this chapter

Secretion of Mucus

Voice not Clear

- Hoarse
- Lost
- Toneless

34. External Throat and Neck:

Throat External

Nape

Cervical and Submaxillary Glands & Thyroid Gland etc are given in this chapter.

35. Nape and Nape of Neck:

This chapter includes only the sides Left and Right.

36. Chest:

Misplaced rubrics include

Palpitation

Heart's action intermittent

- Tremulous
  Milk Bad
- Increased
- Diminished

37. Back:

Scapulae

Dorsal region

Lumbar and sacral region

Coccyx

And finally sides

- Left and Right are given

38. Upper Extremities:

It include

Shoulder

Axilla (in kent's Repertory it is included under the chapter Chest)

Upper Arm

Forearm

Hand

Palm

Fingers

Nails

Shoulder Joint

Elbow

Wrist

Bones of upper extremities in general Sides- Left and right.

39. Lower Extremities:

Loins (Region of Hips) – Another rubric Loin is given under the External Abdomen Chapter, but here it is specified.

Other rubrics include

Nates

Thigh

Leg below knee

Tibia

Calf

Tendo Achillis

Heel

Back of Foot

Sole

Toes

Nails

Joints of Lower Extremities in General

Hip-Joint

Knee

Knee- Hollow of

Patella

Ankle

Toe – Joint

Bones of Lower Extremities in General

Left &

Right sides

3. Sensations

It include rubrics related to various Complaints also, hence Boger has renamed this chapter as Sensations and Complaints in General.

Certain important rubrics in this chapter include

Apoplexy

Burns

Carphology

Carried desires to be (might have been given under Mind)

Chlorosis

Clothing Intolerance of

Cold tendancy to take

Consumption in General

Convulsions

Cracking of Joints'

Cyanosis

Dislocations

Dropsy Externally & Internally

Emaciation

External Parts, Drugs affecting

Faintness

Frozen limbs

Haemorrhage from Internal Parts

Hysteria

Immobility of Affected Parts

Indurations

Inflammations Externally, internally

Internal Parts, Drugs affecting

Labor – like Pains (same rubric can be seen under the Chapter Sexual organs)

Looked at, Aversion To Being (Misplaced – Might be given Under the Chapter Mind)

Motion Aversion, To (")

Mucus secretions Increased

Obesity

Pain Jumping from Place to Place

Paralysis – One sided

Polypus

Reeling

Restlessness

Retraction of Soft Parts

Scurvy

Sit Inclination to

Sprain from lifting

Ulcerative pain Externally

-      Internally

Washing, Dread of {These two rubrics may be more suitable if Water, Dread of Whirling { given in the Mind Chapter}

Glands:

The main rubrics include ;

Atrophy

Indurations

Inflammation

Injuries

Swelling

- like knotted cords

    Suppuration

    Ulcers

- cancerous

Bones:

It includes the following important rubrics

Healing of Broken Bones

Inflammation

Caries

- of periosteum

Necrosis

Softening

Skin:

Blood Sweating

Chilblains

Color, Yellow

Corns

- Horny

- Sensitive

    Desquamation

    Eruptions

- Carbuncles

- Chicken Pox

- Furuncle

- Itch (Scabies)

- Suppressed

- With Maggots

- Measles

- Pimples

- Small-Pox

- Zoster

- Condylomata

- Cysts,Sebaceous

    Extravasations

    Gangrene

    Hair of Head Falls Out

- Beard

- Moustache

    Nails , Brittle

    Sore, Becomes (Decubitus)

    Stings of Insects

    Tetter in General (herpetic)

- Ring Worm

    Ulcers, Varicose

    Wounds in General

- Old Wounds Break Out

4. Sleep:

This chapter include sleep in general, positions during sleep, and dreams. The last two are given as separate chapters. Important rubrics to note are;

Yawning

Sleep Comatose

Sleep Somnambulistic

Sleep Unrefreshing

Symptoms Causing Sleeplessness

Dreams Pleasant, of Gold (this should be interpreted as dreams of money)

Dreams of Love (= dreams Amorous)

5. Fever

From the page 250 to 252 the top heading is circulation, from page 253 it is changed to Fever.

This chapter includes

Circulation

Chilliness in general

Heat

Coldness in general

Shivering in general

Sweat in general

Compound Fevers in General

Though Circulation is given as a separate chapter it is included under the Fever Chapter. The old Edition contain these seven sub- sections.

Circulation Chapter include the following rubrics

Blood, Anaemia

Blood vessels inflammation

- Varicose

Pulse, intermittent

- Irregular
- More rapid than the beat of heart
- Slower than the beat of heart

Chill chapter contains

Chilliness One sided

Chilliness with Thirst

Chilliness Symptoms during Chill (concomitants of Chill stage)

Heat Chapter include

Heat without thirst

– With inclination to uncover

– With dread of uncovering

– Associated symptoms (concomitants)

Sweat includes

Sweat on one side

– Bloody

– Exhausting

– Odorous

Sweat with associated Symptoms
In compound fevers occurrence of different

stages of fever is given. For example;
Chill then heat

Heat then chill

Chill internally and heat externally

Heat alternating with sweat

Concomitants of Fever are given as
Before fever

During fever

After fever

The chapter ends with

Febrile Symptoms – Left side

– Right side

6. Alterations of the state of Health

a. Aggravation

First the time modalities are given, specific time modalities are not given. It include the following rubrics

During Day

Morning

Forenoon

At noon

Afternoon

Evening

Night

Other important rubrics include

Arsenic fumes

Bathing

Biting Teeth together

Blowing nose

Breakfast after

Breathing

Burns

Brushing Teeth

Change of Weather

Children Especially, Remedies

Clear Weather

Climateric during

Closing Eyes

Cloudy weather

Clutching anything

Coition during & after

Cold in General

Combing hair

Drinkers, for Hard (old Topers)

Driving in a Wagon

Eructation

Eruptions after Suppression of

Excitement, Emotional

- Contradiction

- Fright– grief and sorrow

- Mortification

- V exation

  Exertion, Mental

– Physical

Exertion of Vision

Fasting

Food and Drink

- Alcoholic stimulants in general

- Beans and peas

- Farinaceous

- Milk

- Tobacco

Grasping anything tightly

Hang down, letting limbs

Hiccough

House in the

Hunger

Inspiration

Labor, manual

Lifting

Loss of Fluids

Lying – in – women

Measles after

Moon, New

– full

– waning

Moonlight

Music

Narcotics

Narrating Her Symptoms

Nursing Children

Odors, Strong

Pregnancy

Pressure of clothes

Rest

Rising Up

Room Full of People

Sexual Excesses

Shaving

Sitting, when

Sleep, before

- At the Beginning of

- During

- After

Smoke

Society

Squatting down

Stone Cutters, for

Stooping

Stranger, when among

Sun, in The

Swallowing

Sweat, During

- After

- Suppression of

Talking

Touch

Uncovering

Vertigo During

Vomiting

Warmth in General

Water (and Washing)

Wet applications

Wet, getting

Wet Weather

Wind

Women, For

Writing

Yawning

b.   Amelioration

Important rubrics to be referred are

Attention paying

Carrying the child in the arms

Crossing Limbs

Exerting Mind

Fasting (Before Breakfast)

Flatulent Emissions

Haemorrhage

Inspiration

Loosening Clothes

Mesmerism

Motion of Affected Parts

Scratching

Sleep During & After

Swallowing

Walking in Open air

Some rubrics does not contain medicines, their reference is given in brackets. They are asked to refer in the Aggravation chapter- among the rubrics with opposite meaning.

For example;

Cloudy Weather (see Agg. Clear Weather)

Cold, in the (see Agg. Warmth in General)

Damp Weather (See Agg. Dry Weather)

Food and drinks, Hot (see Agg. Food and Drinks, Cold)

Hang Down, Letting Limbs (See Agg. Raising Affected Limbs)

Silence (see Agg. Noise)

Society (See Agg. Alone, When)

Warm (see Agg. Cold, Becoming)

7.   Relationship of remedies

Uses   of   relationship   chapter
In the earlier editions the name of this chapter was Concordance of Remedies. This chapter contains relationship of 141 Medicines.

1.   It can be used for studying the relationship of remedies at various levels- mind, parts, sensation, modalities .

2.   It is helpful for finding out the second prescription

3.   In certain cases a deep acting medicine cannot be given eventhough indicated, so as to avoid unwanted precipitation of adverse symptoms.

Method of working

When the indicated medicine has helped a little and when there is no further improvement this section can be referred to find out a close medicine which would help the patient.

Under that medicine(first prescription) refer the sub-heading which could be the main complaint of the patient and use it as first rubric. Next take the Mind and all other sub headings one after another. The first rubric can taken as an eliminating rubric.

Those medicines with higher marks (3,4,5 marks) are taken for further repertorisation. If it is a case of tonsillitis –' Glands' are taken as the first rubric. Subsequent rubrics are referred. After examination process the medicine with maximum number of marks are selected as second prescription.

Advantage of TPB

1. It is based upon the concept of complete symptom- location, sensation, modality, and concomitant.

2. It follows more or less an anatomical schema which is helpful for finding the rubrics.

3. By applying the 'Doctrine of analogy' rubric can be completed, even though there is lack of any of the four parts of the symptom.

4. Five gradations of medicines are one of the unique contribution of Boenninghausen.

5. This repertory has given more importance to concomitant symptoms than Kent's repertory.

6. Modalities are given under separate section. Ameliorations are also given more importance than Kent's repertory.

7. This repertory is useful in working out cases which are full of particulars and which contain few mental generals and physical generals. Cases manifested by pathological changes and objective symptoms can better dealt by BTPB.

8. Rubrics are given in simple language.

9. Chapter 'relationship of remedies' is helpful for finding the second prescription.

10. The sides of the body are given importance, they are mentioned in location chapter.

11. The extremities are divided into upper and lower which is helpful for finding the rubrics very easily.

Disadvantage of BTPB

1. It deals with only 342 remedies. Boenninghausen's original edition contained 126 remedies. Allen dropped 4 remedies (Angustra, Magnetis Polus Articus, Magnetis Polus Australius, Magnetis Poli Umbo) and added 220 remedies.

2. The rubrics given in the book are not many in number.

3. Many of the rubrics lack important medicines-desire for salt – Natrum mur is not mentioned.

4. Mind section contains only 18 rubrics under 'mind' and 17 rubrics under intellect. These rubrics are too general and can only be used as reference.

5. The concept that a symptom that refers to a part may be predicated of the whole man (Doctrine of analogy) is not correct under many circumstances.

6. Though prime importance is given to the concomitants there is no separate chapter for them.

7. Even though this book has undergone many modifications and editions there are many defects in the construction and compilation.

8. – Internal head ends on page 26 , again starts on page 29.

9. – External head ends on page 29 , again starts on page 30.

10. Rubrics that might have been placed under ' sensations' are given under 'parts of the body'- Toothache under teeth, stopped feeling in ears.

11. There is no fixed arrangements of rubrics.

12. The relationship section deals with only 141 remedies.

13. There are many misplaced rubrics- Vertigo-is given in intellect,Perineum is given in chapter stool.

14. Different sensations are given specifically , but in practice many patients do not specify their sensations.

15. This book lacks information about Sarcodes and Nosodes.

IMPORTANCE OF CONCORDANCE CHAPTER

In the **concordances Boenninghausen's keen** , observant mind noticed that there exist a relationship among the medicines. He incorpaorated a chapter on this, in his TPB towards the end with title "Concordance of remedies". Dr Boenninghausen's own experience and the study of remedies had helped him to compile the "Relationships of Remedies", which would in fact render important service to the system. In the earlier edition of the book, he referred to this chapter as concordance of Remedies , but Allen gave it more comprehensible title 'relationship of Remedies'. He discusses the relationship of remedies under the headings – Mind, Localities,Sensations, glands, bones, skin,sleep and dreams, blood , circulation, fever, aggravation, other remedies, antidote, and inimical/injurious.

In the repertory of antipsoric remedies there were some sections which were later changed in his therapeutic pocket book. In the Repertory of antipsoric medicines there were 45 chapters , the chapter concordance were not included. Aggravations and ameliorations are given at the end of each chapter. The section Mind and intellect had the name mind and soul. All these changes are because of application of doctrine of analogy and doctrine of complete symptoms.

Construction of the chapter

Number of   Medicines in the the relationship part is 142 starting from the aconite to zincum. Gradation is same that of repertory section, ie, 5grades.remedy in parenthesis are for the critical evaluation.later many authors have not considered this last grade remedies. The chapter on Relationship of remedies is divided in to sections- each sections being devoted to a remedy, in alphabetical order Each of these remedy section sub divided in to rubrics, as are all general sections in this book , but in this chapter we find the rubrics are not particularized as symptoms, but generalized symptom groups. Each remedy has 12 subsections which correspond to the general section of the first part of TPB. Subsections include

- Mind
- Localities
- Sensations
- Glands
- Bones
- Skin
- Sleep and dreams
- Blood . circulation and fever
- Aggravations: time and circumstances

To this section added 3 additional rubrics like o

- Other remedies
- Antidotes
- Injurious

The one that is always present bears the title is *other remedies. Other remedies* are those , which have a general relationship to the remedy under consideration and not only to the specific subsection. Of the other two rubrics which occationally appear , *antidotes* and *injurious* are easily comprehended. He used the word "noxious" instead of injurious. This section of book is far from being as complete as the other chapters.

Dr Boenninghausen wrote "for myself, material medica pura is the most indispensible works of homoeopathy, thus concordance has been extreme importance , not only for the recognition of the genius of the remedy , but also for testing and making sure of its choice and fore judging of sequence of the various remedies especially in chronic diseases. Clinical relationship does exist on a definite doctrine but it is obscured at present."

Relationship of remedies is an important consideration in second prescription, when the symptomatology has changed or when in the treatment of chronic case , some acute trouble has cropped up. A knowledge of the relationships of superficial and antipsoric remedies or those of the nosodes is great help in prescribing the follow up medicines.

The chapter Relationship of Remedies has the following uses / Adaptability of the chapter relationships of remedies

- It can be used for studying the relationship o remedies at various levels – mind, parts, sensations, modalities

- Helps to find out close running medicine, which can be thought in future follow up.

- To find out second medicine, ie, first one (though indicated) doesn't meet with expectation in a given period of time

- In order to avoid unwanted precipitation of adverse symptoms, when a deep acting remedy is given, in those cases analogous can be found out.

E.g. – in case of an advanced tuberculosis

To elicit the chronic to acute relationship of remedies

- To find cyclical or sequential relationship

- Helps us to study various relationship of remedies .

- Cases where the outstanding complaint of the pateint were related bones , glands ,skin etc... we can select remedies from rubrics , under remedy that served well at first in the acute case

- It helps in the study of comparative MM- the symptomatology in a patient move in closely related field rather extend in to totally unrelated one, as the final choice being as always confirmed by reference to materia

This concept of relationship of remedies and its reportorial analysis is the unique contribution made by Dr Boenninghausen in the promotion of scientific prescribing in homoeopathic practice. He evaluated closely similar remedies and elaborated the unique concept of remedy relationships. It establishes the relationship between acute and deep acting constitutional remedies. Antidotal and inimical relationship are largely of use in the clinical practice , so also the so called "cycles". We can use relationship of remedies in above conditions such as *antidote, complementary, cognate , change of remedy, change of plan of treatment.*

The relationship of remedy indirectly a probable sequence of changes in the susceptibility also. Boenninghausen's critical study of symptomatology in homoeopathic materia medica and wide spread clinical experience are reflected in the section of relationship of remedies in therapeutic pocket book. This knowledge grown with additions made subsequently by Boger, Knerr,Kent, Hering and others.

The concepts relates similar picture to each other ,relates the main picture to sector wise or miasm wise, projects sequential changes likely to occur in the future under the influence o the selected remedy, relates the main picture to the partial expressions of nosodes as anti- miasmatic drugs and also stresses antidotal and inimical relationships derived purely from clinical experience.

Working method

Introduction to TPB dealt with a case – of simple fever and cold in a child of 3 years, the remedy suited were belladonna, but belladonna failed to control temperature of 105 degree centigrade. So the case was analysed by the chapter on relationships under the remedy belladonna. Only the remedies ranking 3,4,5 under the mind were taken and the other rubrics under belladonna were checked against them. So that we can find the drug with maximum mark is related very closely to that condition. In this we will get PULS as most valuable related remedy.

Different types of relationship of remedies . they are -

Family relationship – derived by similarity of origin(eg- OPHIDia group have similar tendencies like haemorrhagic iathesis, constrictions etc).

Concordant relationship – marked similarity in action though dissimilar in origin, they may follow each otherwell (aloes and sulphur – both have abdominal plethora and portal congestion).

Complementary—one drug completes a cure which the other begins but is unable to complete. The complementary drug completes the work of a given remedy.(E.G., BRY and RHUS). There are acute and chronic complementary. *Cognates* are the complementary remedies in series (e.g. – Bry- sulph-calc carb- tub).

Antidotes – medicine given to counter act a poison or disease. In homoeopathy it is the medicine given to counteract, minimize,or moderate the over action or undesired effects of a drug either during proving or during the therapeutic use. Symptom similarity is the basis of antidotel relationship of medicines.

Inimical- -drugs although resembling each other apparently, will not follow one another with any satisfaction. They seems to mix up the case. The more closely similar the remedies , the greater the similarity of their symptoms, the greater risk of antagonism between themans more certain the second remedy will injure the case.

Intercurrent— needed after a remedy, for the repetition of the first one with much advantage. Usually they have a complementary relation to first one. (nat mur will not be repeated without an intercurrent. (Dr. Hahnemann).

Other authors said about relationship of remedies

Dr Hahnemann said in the aphorism 249, he suggest, "if the aggravation be considerable(after a medicine), be first partially neutralized as soon as possible by *an antidote* before giving the next remedy chosen more accurately according to similarity of action." Also he says, "subsequent doses often removes, curatively, some one or other of the symptoms caused by the previous dose" in aphorism 131.

Dr John Henry Clarke – in his clinical repertory. Gives in a tabular form , the chief clinical relations of all remedies in the following headings- *complementary, remedy follows well,remedy is followed well by, compatible remedies, incompatible,remedy antidotes,remedy is antidote by,duration of action.*

Dr Calvin broast Knerr – dealt with different types of drug relationships. Like *antidotes, collaterals,compatible, complementary, inimical, similar .*

Boger BBCR also dealt with relationship of remedies under the chapter the concordance. Arrangement and construction followed from TPB , but the number of remedies in each headings are less and there fore the practical purposes it falls short and cannot complete with TPB.it contain only 125 remedies.

E A farrington – says about , *family relations, concordant relation, complement, antidote, enmity or inimical.*

Dr.Gibson Miller – *complements,remedies that follows well, inimical* – (quoting Kent, says that some remedies areinimical to each other in acute sphere and others inimical only in chronic sphere,) and also about *antidotes.*

Dr H A Robberts *Complimentary, antidote, neutral, remedies with lesser degrees of similarity, inimical, succession of remedies*

Dr R E Dudgeon – *antidote ,(antidotarial influence of medicines up on one another depends solely up on the homoeopathuc principle")*

Dr J T Kent – *chronic remedy* – (Eg – calc is the neutral chronic of bell and RHUS),*complimentary, inimical, antidote.*

Dr Stuart close – days about the *antidotes,* they are divided in to 3 classes, physiological/ dynamical, chemical and mechanical.

Dr H L Chitkara – *compliments, antidotes ,remedies follow well ,inimical or incompatible,antidotes to,*

Dr CONSTANTINE HERING –*complementary to, incompatible to, compatible to, antidotes.*

Dr Elizabeth wright hubbard – *Complementary,* 3 types – plain relationship,acute compliments of chronic remedies, remedies in series., *incompatible,vegetable analogues/ chemical analogues, botanical relationships.*

Dr J BenedictD' castro – *harmonious* means most similar one are complementary and they antidote the bad effects, *neutral,* an dinimical.

Dr P Sankaran – *complements, remedies that follow well, inimical, antidotes, collaterals* (They are similar in their symptom picture but they are noy related in any way).

Dr Garth Boericke – *family relations, antidotal relationship, concordant or compatible, complementary, inimical.*

Dr B K Sarkar – *Complementary , concordant remedies.* (He says that the concordant have marked similarity in action , although they belong o different or natural groups. This group includes complementary remedies and remedies which follows well.), *antidotal remedies, inimical remedies, incompatible, collateral, remedies which follows well.*

Changes made by H.C. Allen in BTPB:

1) Allen dropped out 4 remedies to the original of 126 remedies of BTPB and added 220 new remedies , thus total became 342.

2) Allen gave the 7th chapter of "Concordance" a more comprehensible name i.e, "Relationship of Remedies".

Changes made by H.A. Roberts in BTPB:

1) He added new 20 remedies to Allen's edition and thus total number of remedies became 362.

Life sketch of Dr CM Boger(1861-1935)

Dr. Cyrus Maxwell Boger was born as the son of Prof.Cyrus and Isabelle Maxwell Boger on 1861. He received his early education in the public school of Lebanon Pa and graduated from the Philadeiphia college of medicine. He later studied at Hahnemanns Homoeopathic college in Philadeipia and qualified himself as a homoeopath. He was as American homoeopath of German origin and was a contemporary of Dr. Kent.

Dr. Boger became widely known through a large number of learned contributions to the Homoeopathic literature. His authorship of several medical books, his repertory construction, translation of several medical books from notable German authors and his indefatigable labor in research made him universally recognized as an author of considerable eminence.

Some important literary works of Dr. Boger are

- Transactions of the original Repertory of Antispsorics (Systematic Alphabetic Repertory Of Homoeopathic Materia Medica)- 1899-1900.

- Boenninghausens characteristics & Repertory – 1905.

- Synoptic key to Materia Medica – 1915.

- Times of remedies and Moon Phases – 1931.

- General Analysis - 1924

- Studies in Philosophy and healing -1931

- Additions to Kents Repertory

- Translation of TPB - 1900

- Card Repertory – Boger Boenninghausen slips - 1924

These works made him universally recognised as an author of considerable eminence. Probably there has never been a more through student of Boenninghausen than later Dr. CM Boger. Perhaps the greatest piece of literature left by Dr. Boger is Boenninghausen's characterstic and Repertory based on the original Repertory of antipsoric remedies but brought up to date and more valuable by the addition of more rubrics remedies and also by the addition of synoptic Materia Medica as one section of the book.

Dr: Boger aged 74 passed away on 2nd sept 1935 after as illness lasting 2 weeks.

H/o and Evolution of Boger's Repertory. During the later part of 19th century , with the emergence of Kents repertory the applications of Boenninghausen Therapeutic pocket book was relegated to the back stage. Boger was an ardent follower of Boenninghausen's school of philosophy which in his view was much closer to Hahnemannian concept of disease understanding. Dr: Boger was a prolific writer on the use of repertories who was at ease with both Kents and Boenninghausen's school of philosophy. The construction and informations based in Kent's repertory also impressed him. So he embarked on the mission of achieving and integration of the information present in these two reportories.

While Dr: Boger was practicing in US he understood the difficulties faced by the practitioners of his days in finding out a similimum from the Materia Medica in the shortest possible time. Finding that the practitioners had to depend on the existing faulty translations of the Repertory of Antipsorics he took up the task of translating it in 1899. While doing this translation he was further convinced that Boenninghausen's basic principles plan and construction were sound and the book was comprehensible and practicable. He was also aware of the difficulties faced by practitioners while using Therapeutic pocket book as well as the criticisms leveled against its principles and methodology.

So he took up the work of rewriting Boenninghausen's Repertory by adding new chapters, new rubrics and new medicines. Thus he modified chapter of Therapeutic pocket book by adding modalities and concomitant at the end of each chapter. The outcome was a more useful work and was published by Boericke and Tafel in 1905. Even after the publication of the Ist edition Boger continued to work on the Repertory. But he could not survive to see the publication of the 2nd edition of his Repertory. Later the manuscripts were published posthumously with the assistance of his wife by Roy & company in 1937. This can be considered as the 1st Indian edition of Bogers Repertory.

2nd Indian edition was also brought forth by Roy & Company in 1952. 3rd Indian edition was published by B.Jain after 20 years in 1972. All the present edition are reprints of the 2nd edition published in 1937.

A. BOGER BOENNIGNHAUSENS CHARACTERISTICS AND REPERTORY

Full name of the book is Boenninghausen's characteristics and Repertory.

Characteristics includes the 'characteristic symptom of Boenninghausen translated by Boger for the first time. They are the same characteristic symptom as seen in other Materia Medicas. This materiamedica part deals with symptomatology of each remedy and permits ready reference to Materia Medica. Boger's translations of original rubric from German to English has been stated to be more accurate than that of Allen.

Classification

It comes under the classification of LOGICAL UTILITARIAN TYPE. This Repertory is based on the logic of particulars to generals especially on pathological generals & complete symptom based on the doctrine of INDUCTIVE LOGIC.

Source books

Source book Materia Medica part

- Boenninghausen's characteristics translated by Boger for the first time.
- Whooping – cough – homoeopathic Treatment of whooping Cough in its Various forms published by Boenning hausen in 1860.
- Homoeopathic Domestic Physician in Brief Therapeutic Diagnosis-1853.
- Therapeutic Hints from the Aphorisms of Hippocrates.
- Symptom Text of Intemittent fever.

- Aided remedies are added at the end of remedy which are the results of long years of observation by Boenninghausen.

Philosophical background of Boger Boenninghausen characteristics and repertory

Boenninghausens pioneering work was in great use during the second half of the 19th century because it was the only work of its kind available to the practitioners. With the publication of kents repertory it receded to the back stage. Consequently BH's work as well as his principles were over looked. Boger creditably resuscitated Boenninghausen by refining and enriching the fundamentals and recasting the sturcture and methodology. Boger subscribed to the principle of totality of symptom which was originally given by Hahnemann.

His work Boenninghausen characteristic and repertory is based on the following fundamental concepts.

1. Doctrine of complete symptom
2. Doctrine of pathological generals
3. Doctrine of causation and time
4. Clinical rubrics
5. Evaluation of remedies
6. Fever totality
7. Concordances

While taking the case history of all symptoms of the patient, it may not be complete in terms of sensations, locations, modalities and concomitants. Boenninghausen noted these deficiencies in proving also where the provers falls to narrate all the symptom completely.

1. Doctrine of complete symptom

A complete symptom to one which consists of sensation location & modalities. During case taking some symptoms may also be noticed in relation to time before during or after the main complaint. These may not be always having any direct pathological relation to the main complaint Boger got the idea of complete symptom from BH's method of erecting totality but Boger improved the idea by relating sensations and modalities to specific parts. In Bogers Repertory complete symptoms are well arranged and it is seldom necessary to do grand generalisation regarding sensations and modalities.

Concomitants are also given greater importance. They typify the individual reactions and they corresponds to the strange rare and peculiar symptoms of Hahnemann. Common concomitants are unimportant unless they are present in an extraordinary degree.

The most important concomitants are

- Those which are rarely found combined with the main affection, hence also Infrequent under the same condition in proving.
- Those concomitants which belong to another sphere of action of main complaint.
- Those concomitants which belong the distinctive marks of some drugs even if they have never been noted in the proceeding relation before.

2. Doctrine of pathological generals.

In addition to complete symptom Boger also gave importance to general changes in tissues and parts of body. Pathological changes tells us the state of whole body and its changes in relation to the constitution. Pathological generals are expressions of the person which can be known by the study of changes at the tissue level. Some constitutions are prone to some pathological changes in some parts of the body. This common changes in different tissues show the behaviour of the whole constitutions which is important to understand the individual.

3. Pathological generals can be

Structural alterations in tissues organs and systems pertaining to man as a whole. A particular sensation or a local pathology becomes a physical general sensation or a pathological general when interpreted in the light of underlying constitutional state predictive of a generalised disturbance in human economy as. Psycho-physio-pathologic basis.

Eg: pain in heels /Tendo Achilles, uric add diathesis painful sensitive soles, gouty/rheumatic state or sensitive/hysterical/neurotic subject.

Miasmatic background interpretation.

- A solitary want or mole -sycotic
- Localised patch of eczema-psoric
- Fistula in Ano-syphillitic miasm
- Bone pains at night- syphilitic miasm.

Constitution /Diathesis.

Re-current Epistaxis-Heamorrhagic diathesis.

Recurrent boils, delayed healing of wounds and ulcers, easy suppuration-diabetic state.

Structural alterations common to 2 or more than two location.

Dicharge, Acidity, Excoriation, redness, cracks, Fissuses, Acridity can be can be taken in a still wider context as to include the mind -Acrid mind.

General Locations eg: Glands, skin-folds, flexures, Glands, bends, angles-mouth, corners, canthi, sphincters mucus membranes.

Discharges when common to 2 or more Locations-colour, odour& consistency. Degenerative changes in many location Atrophy & emaciation.

Doctrine of Causations & Time

In Boger's hierarchy of evaluating symptoms He gives more importance to causation & general modalities. In his synoptic key he emphasises that while taking the case we should first try to elicit the evident cause and course of sickness and all which now to interfere with the patients comfort. So according to Boger causation and Time are more definite and reliable in cases as well as in medicines.

Every chapter in his Repertory is followed by sub chapters on Time, Aggravation, Ameliorations and concomitants. Section on Aggravations contains many causative factors. According to him these causative factors are very useful for finding out the similimum in the shortest possible time. In the chapter choosing the remedy he is giving importance to miasmatic as well as exciting causes. The natural tendency to disease may be due to psora syphillis & sycosis. External cause excite disease principally by means of external impressions when there is a natural predisposition. In some cases it is easy to prescribe upon cause. Eg: sprains fever etc. Causations are very important because if the cause is removed the effect will go by itself.

4. Clinical rubrics

Boger was the first person who appreciated the use of clinical conditions in grouping medicines. Several clinical conditions are mentioned in his Repertory which will help the physician in case of advanced tissue changes where we will not get a clear picture because of poor susceptibility. There rubric will help to arrive at a small group of medicine which can be further narrowed down with the help of modalities. These clinical rubrics can be used when the case is not having any other choice or if the case is lacking in characteristic expressions. This helps mainly in finding out a palliative drug which is suitable in helping to overcome the present crisis.

5. Evaluation of Remedies

Boger followed the same method used by BH. Medicines are graded into 5 rank by the use of different typography such as

- Ist Grade   CAPITALS   5 Marks
- 2nd Grade   Bold   4 Marks
- 3rd Grade   Italics   3 Marks
- 4th Grade   Roman   2 Marks
- 5th Grade   (Roman)   1 Marks

Ist Grade remedies are proved reproved and clinically verified. In the 2nd Grade intensity is slightly lower than the first Grade. Italics / 3 marks remedies are proved & reproved but not clinically verified. Roman – clinically verified but not seen during proving. (Roman) doubtful remedies which needs further study. Apart form these we can find one more gradation Boger's Repertory about which nothing is mentioned. It is indicated as (CAPITALS).

Eg: upper extremities – caries – (ASAF).

6. Fever totality

Is a unique contribution of Boger. This section can be considered as a self contained repertory within the large Repertory. Each stage of fever is completed by Time , Aggravation, Amelioration & concomitant. Fever chapter is almost complete.

7. Concordances

Deals with relationship of 125 remedies. It can be used for studying the relationship of remedies at various levels as mind, parts, sensation and modalities.

Boger's concept ot totality

In the chapter choosing the remedy he emphasised the importance of 7 points given by Boenninghausen. Repertory gives us a group of drugs with similar symptomatologies and from this group final differentiation can be made after considering the individualizing or peculiar symptoms. There individualizing features can be

Changes in personality and temperament (Quis) - This should be noted especially when striking alterations occur. These may sometimes obscure the physical manifestations and these may be corresponding to only a few remedies. The expressions of the moral and mental activities affords the best for the choice of medicines in mental affections.

Nature and peculiarities of the disease (Quid) - The nature of the disease and virtues of drugs should be thouroghly known before we can give aid in sickness. Knowledge of disease or diagnosis helps to exclude all medicines which donot correspond to the nature of the disease.

Diagnosis will not help us much for the sure selection of the similar remedy.

Seat of disease(Ubi) :Almost every drug acts definitely upon certain parts of the organism. Whole body io not equally affected even in local or general disease some drugs affect (RT) side some (Lt) side and some diagonally. So in order to cure it is essential to ascertain the seat of action. eg: The specific curative powers of sepia in fatal joint abscesses of fingers and toes to extraordinarily conclusive evidence upon thio point , for they differ from similar gatherings only in locations and remedies so suitable for abcess elsewhere remains ineffectual here. Here he says that if the diagnosis of our time were known to Hahnemann he would have localised remedies moreaccurately than simply saying right,left etc.

Concomitants (Quibus Auxillus) – While selecting the simillimum concomitants should be given much importance. Common or well known accompaniments are unimportant unless they are present in an extraordinary degree or appear in a singular manner. The most important concomitant symptoms are

- Those which are rarely found combined with the main affection hence also infrequent under the same condition in proving.
- Those concomitant which belong to another sphere of disease than that of the main one.Eg: cough > paasing flatus
- Those symptoms which bear the distinctive marks of some drug even if they have never been noted in the proceeding
- Relation before.

Important concomitants may sometimes out rank the symptoms of the main disease and may help in the selection of the simillimum. These symptoms may give individuality to the totality and are the same characteristic symptoms which Hahnemann called striking extraordinary and peculiar. When the concomitant and main complaint presents with the same modality it will become more important.

Cause (Cur) – Disease causes can be either Internal or external. Internal diseases arise from internal disposition which is highly susceptible. These are due to uneradicated miasms of psora, syphillis and sycosis. When not due to these they are due to remenants and sequate of acute affections, due to drug disease poisoning etc or due to combination of drug disease with the other which is very difficult to treat and in which cases antipsoric remedies will be very effective. In many of the acute diseases rapid and durable cures can be effected by the administration of antipsortc remedies.In the treatment of many diseases the best selected remedy is often ineffectual unless preceded by a suitable antipsoric, antisyphillitic or antisycotic. While dealing with drug diseases drugs given should be properly ascertained and treated.

Drugs diseases are generally compound & will not show a clear picture hence the knowledge of contents of former prescription to necessary. In some cases it is very easy to find the cause and helps to find a similar remedy eg: burns, sprains etc: But if different cauaes can produce the same condition the choice may become difficult-
Eg: Common cold – After sweating
– By exposure of a part
– By drenching in rain

Dr. Boger to giving much important to the causative modalities.

So without knowing the cause, the correct homoeopathic remedy cannot be selected.

Modalities According to situation and circumstances (Quomodo) – Modalities are the modifiers of characteristics. All well proved drugs manifests common symptom of many drugs but their modalities may be differing. Modalities must be specialised eg: If motion generally aggravates we should note the different kinds of motion as whether they arise during commencement or are continued etc. General modalities and particular modalities are important. Cravings and aversions to various food materials furnishes important points in deciding the remedy. According to Dr: Boger when symptom are pointing to one particular remedy and if modalities don't agree it will not be indicated and we will have to search for another remedy having same or similar modalities.

Time Modalities (Quando) – Time factors are equally important as aggravations and ameliorations. Here two important things to be noted are the periodical return of symptoms after a shorter or longer period of quiescence. In these types there may be some special or accidental causes such as menstural disturbances, seasonal or temperature influences etc.

E.g. : Fever every 14 days Convulsions during menses.

The hour of days when the disease is better or worse.

These are of much greater importance because we can find these features in many disease and we can find this in many proving so these are peculiar and are qualified.

E.g.: time modalities of cough, diarrhoea etc. unless they are clear and decided (iike hell & lyco at 4-8pm) or return at exactly the same hour (Antc, Ign , Sab) they are unimportant.

It is easy to select the right remedy after a picture of disease complete in respect and fully meeting all requirements has been drawn up then to obtain the materials for such a picture and costruct it for one's self.

Evaluation of symptoms:

Apart from the above mentioned 7 points Dr: Boger appreciated the use of time factors , causative modalities.

Pathological generals and tissue changes to understand the case.

Causative modality Mental & physical – fear, Excitement Physician should try to elicit the evident cause and course of sickness down to the latest symptom. To this add all things which now seems to interfere with the patients comfort.

Modalities

Modalities or natural modifiers of the sickness should be then ellicited. The most vitally important of such influences are Time temperature, openair , posture, Being alone, Motion,sleep ,Eating and Drinking ,Touch, Pressure, Discharges etc.

Mental state

Important point to be noted here are the presence of irritability, sadness fear placidity etc. Mind is given adequate importance and for selecting a drug it becomes imperative that the remedy

selected is always in agreement with the mind. The interdependence of mental and physical states is so great that we can never afford to overtook it entirely.

Sensations

Estimate the patients own description of his sensation. Always ascertain whether any of the following primary sensations are present like Burning, Cramping , Cutting. Bursting , soreness , Throbbing and Thirst. Others may also be present but presence of any one of these may often overshadows them.

Entire objective Aspect or expression of the sickness This Includes facial expresion Demeanor, Nervous Excitability, Restlessness Facial expression, Torpor , colour & odour of secretions, sensibility and any abnormal colouring.

Parts affected or locations must be determined. This will be more helpful in reaching the diagnosis.

By going over the above rubrics in this manner the contour of the disease picture will be clearly outlined and will point clearly towards the similar remedy. The actual differntiating factor may belong to any these rubrics. From these it is very clear that Boger has given importance to causation modalities, concomitants , General sensations & Pathology and location to given last importance in the order of hierarchy.

Diagrammatical representation of evaluation

MODALITIES – Causative Modalities, Time, Temperature weather, open air, posture , motion, eating and drinking, sleep. if alone, pressure, touch, discharges. MIND – Irritability, sadness, fever, placidity.

SENSATION – Burning, Cutting, Cramping, Bursting, Soreness, throbbing, Thirst.

OBJECTIVE ASPECT Demeanor, Restlessness, Nervous Excitability, Facial Expression, Torpor, Secretions , Colour, Odour.

PART AFFECTED – Organ, Right, Left.

Plan and construction of BBCR
Having found certain difficulties in the day to day use of TPB Boger tried to modify the structure and content of the book by adding many medicine and rubrics drawn from his own experience and other sources. Thus the book has undergone a vast change but its basic principles have remained unchanged.

The book consists of:
Materia Medica Part

Repertory Part

Before these two sections book contains
A Foreword written by Dr:HA Roberts in 1938 He emphasises that the works of Boenninghausen are the most comprehensive in logic , philosophy and applicability of the early writers perhaps with the single exception of works of Hahnemann. He stresses this point by noting that even though Hahnemann compiled a brief index to remedies and Jahr preceded Boenninghausen's publication of Rep of Antipsoric remedies it was Boenninghausen who first evaluated remedies in relation to individual symptom

and it was he who first introduced the Relationship of remedies to the individual case. Boenninghausen evolved the doctrine of concomitants which he believed to be of peculiar and characteristic value.

Many criticism have been raised against Boenninghausen's TPB on the ground that there has been no differentiation between general & particular modalities. But in this like its predecessor The Repertory of Antipsorics modalities for each part is assembled at the end of the section of Repertory devoted to that part and a section for general modalities in arranged towards the end of the book.

This book to a valuable addition to the Homoeopathic literature in making available the combined observation and logic of Boenninghausen and the wide and wise observation gathered by Dr.Boger from long year of study & practice.

- Historical sketch of Boenninghausen
- Preface- 2 parts
- Introductory essay about source books
- Notes by Dr: Boger
- On the use of Repertories
- Choosing the Remedy
- Repetition of Dose
- Homoeopathic prognosis
- Index of contents
- Index of medicines in Materia medica part
- Index of chapters in Repertory part

The sections in repertory are given as 53 units but there is a total of 58 chapter because one chapter given as subchapter in index appear as main chapters in the body of the book.

After the Materia Medica and Repertory part towards the end of book there are three more indexes dealing with Word index to Boger Boenninghausen's Rep compiled by S.P Roy.

Word index constitutes 101 pages. Index to main sections / chapters Index to main chapters & subchapters.

Word index arranged chapter wise. The index of the book is excellent and exhaustive which enables even a novice to locate the symptom more readily. In spite of all these the Repertory is lacking in an index of remedies represented in the repertory part.

Later an index was prepared by Dr. Tiwari where he gives the total no: of remedies represented in Repertory to 442. But originally this book contains 489 remedies. Total No of Pages – 1231 pages . which are arranged double coloums.

Arrangement of materia medica part
A total no of 140 medicines are given in the materia medica part in alphabetical order. Each medicine the contents are arranged in Hahnemannian schema i.e from head to foot in each remedy Allied Remedies are given as the last section which list a group of remedies which are related in some way or other with the remedy. In some cases complimentary remedies are included separately.

After all remedies a brief note is given regarding the duration of Action of Remedies where he classifies all remedies into 5 groups as

- Shortest action
- Brief action
- Medium duration of action
- Long acting Remedies
- Very long & deep acting remedies

There are taken from the notes of Hering confirmed by Boenninghausen and it is said that the symptoms which appeared last in the proving are of great value. In a section on important hints 12 observation given by Dr J.T Kent to arranged in a condensed form. In the MM part remedies are graded into 2 i.e italics & ordinary Roman.

Dr: Boger was also impressed by the data presentation in Kents Repertory. He therefore attempted to arrange and improvise the information present in Boenninghausen's repertory as an organised and easily accessible manner. So he presented the data in such a way that a symptom could be repertorised as a unit in the relevant chapter Itself. This was a phenomenal shift from the facility of Boenninghausen's repertory where each element of the symptom had to be repertorised from different sections.

This improvement was accomplished by arranging the relevant sensation, there modifying factors (Agg&Amel) and accompanying symptoms (concomitants) under each locations. Thus the book has undergone a vast change but its basic principles have remain unchanged.

To make this arrangement more comprehensible he differentiated the heading in the 2nd chapter of TPB (parts of body and organs) into distinct headings or separate chapters. While doing this he arranged each location according to Hahnemann's anatomical schema and are given as separate chapters. In this arrangement he followed the pattern adopted by Boennighausen for the construction of Rep of Antipsoric (ie each location followed by sub chapter on <,> and concomitants.) Boenninghausen divided his repertory into seven sections and that plan has been faithfully followed by Boger, In compiling his repertory. Hence the general section in BBCR is same as that of TPB.[But headings like mind & intellect, parts of body and organs etc are lacking in BBCR , instead they appear as separate units. Boger also improved the Repertory by expanding on the mental rubrics. This strategy facilitated its use even in cases where the mental symptoms predominate.

SPECIAL FEATURES OF BBCR:

1) Complete symptoms – The location is followed by the particular sensations, modalities and concomitants, which are lacking in TPB.

2) Diagnostic Rubrics:- There are many diagnostic rubrics given in many chapters with group of medicines mentioned against it which are proved and verified.

3) Pathological Generals:- The pathological generals are useful in repertorization and in selection of simillimum, eg:- Inflammation — Sensations and complaints in general.

4) Rubric- Infant, Affections of:- This is a main rubric given in the chapter of, " Sensations and complaints in general" which is useful in paediatric practice.

5) Constitution:- Different types of constitutions are available in the chapter, "Sensations and complaints in general".

6) Separate concomitants:- This chapter follows modalities in most of the locations. Boger has made it more useful by attaching concomitants to the parts.

7) Fever Chapter: It is most valuable chapter for fever cases. Concomitants in relation to chill, heat and sweat are useful for bedside prescriptions.

8) Cross- Reference:- This subdivision is given at the end of most of the chapters, which is helpful.

9) Mind section: The mind section is large and has some important rubrics which are not even given in Kents repertory.

10) Menstruation Chapter: This is well arranged followed by concomitants in following order

Before menses

At the start of menses

During menses

After menses

LIMITATIONS OF BBCR:

1) Chapter of Concordances contains only 125 remedies, which are less than that of BTPB, and also falls short for repertorization.

2) The construction of this repertory is not uniformly structured as some of the chapters are not completely constructed e.g..Sensorium.

3) Mind chapter though there are many rubrics than Kent but it has less sub rubrics.

4) Even in many chapter there are many rubrics with a very few sub rubrics.

5) Concomitant has not discussed detailly in each & every chapter. E.g. respiration no concomitant for vomiting.

6) Similarly modalities are not mentioned in all the chapter in the end.

7) Extensive particularization of some chapters are done, such as teeth, extremities.

8) Neophytes will find difficulty in using this repertory.

9) There is over generalization of some chapters like sensation & complaints in general, even then it is mostly used for particular symptoms only.

10) A limited number of rubrics re mentioned under many rubrics.

11) Bowel Nosodes are not incorporated.

12) Remedies are very limited comparing to the modern repertories.

13) Though the chapter concordances are very useful due to its limited number of rubrics it has limited use.

14) Boger has used similar rubrics in different sections which creates confusion for the beginners, e.g.. Sensorium,Confusion & mind, confused.

15) Many rubrics have single or a few medicines, e.g.. Mind helpless, openhearted.

16) Nosodes are not represented well.

17) Though it has modalities pertaining to chapter, certain modalities like cough
• No index of drugs pertaining to repertory is given.

CONCLUSION

• No repertory can claim perfection

• BBCR ha some useful feature which Kent repertory doesn't have.

• BBCR is not given the same importance as Kent, except in cases of teachers individual preference. Therefore appreciation of the repertory's utilization suffers due to the an inadequate knowledge.

• Otherwise the limitations that one may expect on a repertory are present here also

• This should not be a deterrent for its use & further refinement.

• It is there fore advisable to cultivate familiarity with more than one repertory & make appropriate entries in the repertory which you constantly use.

• Make it a habit to refer to more than one repertory in every difficult case, & you will soon become a successful prescriber.

B. BOGERS SYNOPTIC KEY

The aim of this book is to simplify and introduce method in to this work, so that the truly Homoeopathic curative remedy may be worked out with greater ease and certainty. For this purpose a combination of the analytical and synoptic methods has been thought best.

A clinical symptom is best obtained by asking the patient to tell his own story, which is then amplified and more accurately defined by eliciting the cause and course of sickness to which he will add all the things which now seem to interfere with the sufferer's comfort & thereby he highlighted the importance of individualization at the level of pathological changes by introducing *pathological generals* in his repertory part.

The natural modifiers of sickness — the modalities, which characterize the symptoms in a case. Those modalities are given much importance than the mentals in this repertory.

A consideration of the mental state comes next in order of importance.

The third step consists of patient's own description of his sensations.

Next in order comes the entire objective or expression of the sickness.

Lastly the part affected must be determined.

The details of the above five points are as follows:

MODALITIES
- Causation. Time. Temp.
- Weather. Open air. Posture.
- Motion. Eating and Drinking.
- Sleep. If Alone. Pressure.
- Touch. Discharges.

MIND
- Irritability
- Sadness.
- Fear.
- Placidity.

SENSATION
- Burning. Cramping
- Cutting. Bursting
- Soreness. Throbbing
- Thirst

OBJECTIVE ASPECT
- Restlessness
- Nervous Excitability
- Facial Expression
- Torpor. Secretions
- Color. Odor

PART AFFECTED
- Organs
- Right
- Left.

The synopsis is intended to make clear the general expression or genius of each remedy and thereby help the prescriber correct his bearings. The scope of its contents is much enlarged by bracketing the most nearly affiliated remedies after some of the more important symptoms; this also helps in making differentiations.

PART ONE:

ANALYSIS - A short repertory containing:
- The periods of aggravation.
- Conditions of aggravation and amelioration
- Generalities i.e. consideration of drug affinities for the entire organism
- Regional repertory

The periods of aggravation includes:
- Periodically
- Morning
- Afternoon
- Evening
- Night

Conditions of aggravation and amelioration includes: E.g.
- Air, cold, dry aggravation
- Anticipations, <
- Ascending <
- Bathing >
- Bed, Getting out of <
- Bending <
- Biting or chewing <
- Bleeding > etc

Generalities includes: E.g.
- Aching

- Acridity
- Albuminous
- Alive sensation
- Ammoniacal odor
- Anaemia, chlorosis
- Aneurism
- Apoplexy
- Associated effects
- Ball, lump, knot etc
- Burns
- Cancer
- Carbuncle etc

Regional repertory includes:
- Intellect
- Mind
- Vertigo
- Head
- External head, Bones and Scalp
- Eyes
- Vision
- Ears
- Hearing
- Nose and Accessory cavities
- Face
- Teeth
- Gums
- Palate
- Tongue
- Mouth and Throat
- Saliva
- Taste
- Appetite
- Aversions
- Thirst

- Cravings and Desires
- Water brash
- Heartburn
- Qualmishness
- Hiccough
- Nausea
- Regurgitation
- Retching and gagging
- Vomiting
- Eructations
- Epigastrium
- Stomach and Abdomen
- External abdomen
- Hypochondriae
- Flatulence
- Groins
- Anus and rectum
- Perineum
- Stool
- Micturition
- Urine
- Sediment
- Urinary organs.
- Genitals
- Male organs
- Female organs
- Sexual impulse
- Menstruation
- Leucorrhoea
- Respiration
- Cough
- Larynx and Trachea
- Voice and speech
- External throat
- Neck
- Chest and Lungs

- External chest
- Axillae
- Mammae
- Nipples
- Heart, Circulation and Pulse
- Back, Spine And Cord
- Scapular region
- Dorsal region
- Lumbar region
- Sacrum
- Upper limbs
- Lower limbs
- Skin
- Sleep
- Chill, Chilliness, Coldness etc
- Heat
- Sweat

PART TWO:

SYNOPSIS — An exposition of the important and characteristic features of the most important remedies of the Homoeopathic Materia Medica, with their physiological spheres of activities, modalities and relationships. It includes **323 remedies**.

PART THREE:

Includes

- Table of the approximate duration of action of remedies
- Complementary remedies
- Antagonistic remedies
- Supplemental reference table i.e. a valuable additional table for ready reference to the reportorial portion in the text

At the end list of remedies and their abbreviations are given which have been used in the repertory. It includes **489 remedies**.

Special features of this synoptic key:

Certain rubrics found in this repertory, which are not available in other common repertories. They are as follows:

Break fast after; eating long after; dinner agg; females agg; direction of sensations; pains, (spread of symptoms like, Here and there); ill or sick feeling; internal affections; irregular effects; loose as if; medicine sensitive to; opening & shutting; reaction violent; rising then falling; stretch impulses to; spare habit; walk impulses to; For the rubric dreams of snakes — Lachesis has not been mentioned in any other repertory.

To select the remedy & regarding posology also has been highlighted in this repertory.

The word concordance means

- i) State of being same heart and mind harmony, ii) arrangement in ABC order of important words used by author or in a book
- 1st used in homoeopathic literature by Boenninghausen in BTPB
- The word concordance was replaced by "Relationship of Remedies" by Allen
- Concordance repertory means repertory based on alphabetic arrangement of symptoms of materia medica i.e indexing symptoms without modifying them

Meaning of concordance:

Agreement, harmony

- An alphabetical arrangement of the principal words in a book or author with a list of passages in which each-occurs
- An alphabetical list of the chief words used in a book or by a writer

The word "concordance" means a state of being of the same heart and mind, a harmony, a harmonious arrangement of the symptoms.

This word was first used in Homeopathy by Boenninghausen in Therapeutic pocket book. The word concordance was replaced by "Relation ship of remedies" in later edition of Allen.

A. KNERR'S REPERTORY OF HERING'S GUIDING SYMPTOMS OF OUR MATERIA MEDICA

Author: Calvin B Knerr . M.D

"This belongs to the Puritan type of repertories, where the symptom of the patient is recorded without much change. This repertory also belongs to the group of concordant repertories.

Other works of the author: Repertory of Headaches.

Published By : Jain Publishing Co .

Contents :

Preface

List of remedies

Chapters:

1. Mind and disposition.
2. Sensorium.
3. Inner head
4. Outer head.
5. Eyes.
6. Ears.
7. Nose.
8. Upper face.
9. Lower face.
10. Teeth and gums.
11. Taste and tongue.
12. Inner mouth.
13. Throat.
14. Desires, aversions, appetite, thirst.
15. Eating and drinking.
16. Hiccough, belching, nausea and vomiting.
17. Scrobiculum and stomach.
18. Hypochondria.
19. Abdomen.
20. Stool and rectum.
21. Urinary organs.
22. Male sexual organs.
23. Female sexual organs.
24. Pregnancy, parturition, lactation.
25. Voice, larynx, trachea, bronchia.
26. Respiration.
27. Cough and expectoration.
28. Inner chest and lungs.
29. Heart, pulse and circulation.
30. Outer chest.
31. Neck and back.
32. Upper limbs.
33. Lower limbs.
34. Limbs in general.
35. Rest, position, motion.
36. Nerves.
37. Sleep.
38. Time.
39. Temperature and weather.
40. Fever.
41. Attacks, periodicity.
42. Locality and direction.
43. Sensations in general.
44. Tissues.
45. Touch, passive motion, injuries.
46. Skin.
47. Stages of life and constitution.
48. Drug relation ship.

Lastly — Index.

Total number of pages - 1232.

PLAN AND CONSTRUCTION :

The order of arrangement, followed in the compilation of this repertory is the one inaugurated by Hahnemann, developed, perfected and used by Hering through out his entire materia medica work viz.: the anatomical or regional division into 48 chapters.

Each chapter is alphabetically divided into sections and rubrics sufficient to allow full scope for analysis of the matter contained there in without destroying consistency as a whole.

The division of the page into double columns is deemed most convenient for the eye and is most advantageous to economy of space.

The section word is repeated down the column in preference to the customary —, which like all marks of abbreviation, ciphers, signs etc are apt to become confusing and are not as space saving as might be supposed.

For eg : Chapter Nose - Coryza

Coryza Acrid

Coryza albuminous etc.

The words right and left, better and worse etc, to avoid possible error, is printed out in full.

The ' rubric word ' or heading to each paragraph, (e.g. - Coryza Acrid :) printed in somewhat bolder and blacker type and followed by a : (colon) applies to each symptom in the paragraph, that is the black letter word is to be mentally repeated for every sentence rounded with a semicolon. It will be observed that the symptoms under each rubric follow in alphabetic order.

E.g.: Coryza Bloody : Act sp, 11 Ailan ......
1 sulp; when blowing

11 calad, carbo acid.

There are four marks of distinction: - 1, 11, **1, 11** have the significance as set down in guiding symptoms.

(I) - the lowest, a single light line, designating an occasionally confirmed symptom.

(II) - a double light line, a symptom more frequently confirmed, or if or but once confirmed strictly in character with the genius of the remedy.

(I) - a single heavy line, symptom verified by cures.

(II) - a double heavy line, symptom repeatedly verified.

These degree marks tallies in the main with the four styles of type used by Boenninghausen in his repertory. (θ) — the Greek "theta" standing between the cured symptom and the pathological condition, or the physiological general state, throughout the guiding symptom, is dispensed with there, mainly for the purpose of economizing space, by enclosing the pathological or physiological term in parenthesis; it is to be remembered that the presence of the term by no means shuts out the usefulness of the symptom in other forms of disease:

-    The perpendicular dotted line, marks observation taken from the old school such as harmonize with our law of cure.

  t   -   toxicological extracts.

  θ   -   symptom observed on the sick only - Pie

-    The hand direction cross reference to related symptoms, diseases and conditions.

The repertory is supplemented by a complete index of localities and terms.

As in the guiding symptoms, so in the repertory; original readings, the words of the prover and the clinician are preserved to the letter, it being thought preferable to retain the most delicate shades of meaning, occasionally even different wordings of the same symptoms, by taking refuge in an extra rubric or cross reference, fuse or commingle in a vague generalization at the sacrifice of individuality.

This repertory is a faithful reproduction of the guiding symptoms, its contents classified and indexed. But it can no way can take the place of the larger work. In a repertory, we have separation by analysis for the purpose of classification and ready reference; in materia medica combination by synthesis to enable us to study drug effects in their grand unity and relationship.

Author also mentions his gratefulness to those who has helped him ti bring the work to completion. Especially to Dr, C Guernsey foe valuable assistance with proofs, to Dr. W. H. Phillip, Messrs, Douty,Ziegler,and Field, his son Bayard and others of his family foe clerical assistance; and lastly to his brother in law - Walter E Hering, under whose experienced and skillful management,aided by his old and reliable foreman Wm. Baetzel, the unusually difficult composition and press work have taken place.

Lastly — abbreviations of 408 drugs given. From Abies Nigra to Zizia aurea.

MERITS OF THE BOOK :

1. Useful as a book of reference, to find the desired symptom together with the indicated remedy.

2. The symptoms are given in their original form without much change.

3. Symptoms arranged in alphabetical order under each chapter.

4. About 408 medicines are dealt within the repertory.

5. There are four grading of symptoms, which helps us to understand the relative importance of drugs in the concerned symptom.

6. Since the cross-reference is given, one symptom can be referred to at more than one place.

7. Additional chapters are given in this book, which are not found in any other book.

For eg : Chapters - Pregnancy, parturition , lactation.

Heart, pulse and circulation. Limbs in general.

Rest, position, motion.

Nerves.

Time.

Temperature and weather.

Attacks, periodicity.

Locality and direction.

Tissues.

Touch, passive motion, injuries. Stages of life and constitution.

DEMERITS :

1. This repertory is not useful for systematic repertorisation of a case.

2. The abbreviations given for the medicines are different from other books.

B. THE CONCORDANCE REPERTORY OF THE CHARACTERISTIC SYMPTOMS OF OUR MATERIA MEDICA - WILLIAM. D.GENTRY

AUTHOR

Author Name: William Daniel Gentry

- Dr. Gentry was against the conventional repertoires of Jahr, Lippe, Boenninghausen in which the provers language was not followed and because of this the theme of the symptoms got changed.

- Published in: 1st edition- 1890 2nd edition- 1892

- Title: Concordance Repertory of the Most Reliable Symptoms Found in the Homoeopathic Materia Medica.

- This is the large concordance repertory of 6 volumes.

- In this repertory the symptoms are arranged in alphabetical order under each chapter.

INTRODUCTION

- In preface author says there is a need it may be truthfully said an urgent demand for repertory which will enable the physician to find quickly and certainly ad desired symptom in the materia medica together with the indicated remedy. The concordance repertory is designed to supply this demand

- The idea which finally gave origin to the work presented itself in the autumn of 1876

- He was looking for particular symptom, i.e "constant dull frontal head ache worse in the temples with aching in ht umbilicus". This made it difficult to find

- After weary search author exclaimed if we only had repertory arranged on the plan of cruden's concordance of the Bible. It would have been necessary only to refer the letter U and under umbilicus, find at once. These massive volumes were the end products of that desire

PLAN AND CONSTRUCTION

ARRANGEMENT OF CHAPTERS:

There are 6 volumes and arrangement of chapter under each volume as follows.

- **VOLUME-1** - Mind and Disposition, Head and Scalp, Eyes, Ears, Nose, Face.(6)

- **VOLUME - 2** - Mouth, Throat, Stomach, Hypochondria. (4)

- **VOLUME - 3** - Abdomen, Anus, Rectum and Stool, Urine and Urinary organs, Male Sexual System. (5) -

- **VOLUME - 4** - Uterus and Appendages, Menstruation and Discharges, Pregnancy and Parturition, Lactation and Mammary Gland. (4)

- **VOLUME - 5** - Voice, Larynx and Trachea, Chest, Lungs, Bronchi and Cough, Heart and Circulation, Skin Sleep and Dreams. (6)

- **VOLUME - 6** - Neck and back, Upper extremities, Lower extremities, Bones and limbs in generals, Nerves, Generalities and Key notes. (6)

RULES ADAPTED FOR THE PREPARATION OF THE WORK

Symptoms qualifying following criteria are included in this repertory

- Selected only more characteristic pathogenetic symptoms
- Included only such clinical symptoms as have been repeatedly verified
- Where 2 or more remedies have the power of producing a similar condition, include them as merely suggestive under the name condition produced

    4. Give the noun, verb, and essential objective in the sentence

- Apart from this in the repertory the author has tried to use the phraseology of materia medica without change. E.g under catamenia there are few drugs, where as under menses many. Because in materia medica only few drugs are given with the word catamenia
- One symptom can be referred at many places. E.g confusion in head, which makes thinking difficult. This can be referred under Head & Scalp and also under Mind
- On the top of page, one side 1st 3 alphabets of the starting rubric in capital bold and the other side is the page number, in the middle, chapter name in italics
- For easy reference in between the rubrics he has given 1st 3 alphabets of succeeding rubric in bold capital (Only in 1st VOL)
- Rubrics are given in roman bold followed by a dot and line
- Rubric are arranged in the alphabetical order

- Sub rubrics too arranged in alphabetical order, but not strictly followed. E.g Angry (p.no-5)
- Before starting with sub rubric 1st alphabet of main rubric given in bold. E.g Anger, Ailment, Anxiety
- Sub rubric which are having the main rubric word in between sentence, will be given as 1st alphabet of main rubric in a small letter. E.g Alone, Leucorrhoea, Anger
- From his clinical experience he has given lot of information under some rubrics. E.g leucorrhoea- Acrid & fetid l. Eucalyp (use locally as disinfectant). Lower extremities- stinging- acute Rheumatism-Acon (also apply cloth saturated with dilution)
- Cross references given immediately after the rubrics in brackets. E.g Neck and Back- extremities (see section on extremities). Neck and Back- Palsy (see Paralysis also action on nerves)
- Clinical symptoms are specified at the end of medicine in brackets. E.g Mind and Disposition – gastric (p.no-55)
- The remedies have reverse action of given rubrics is given in brackets and mentioned reversed at the starting followed by drugs. E.g mind and disposition- gentle. (p.no-55). mind and disposition- passes (p.no-105)
- The remedies in brackets indicated that they have some other related rubric. In some rubrics drugs are given in bracket with also. E.g Humour p.no-62)
- In some rubrics diseases which produces that particular conditions are given in brackets. E.g 6th vol Neck and Back (p.no-145)

- In some rubrics, main rubric given at the end of sub rubric(in small letter with 1st alphabet).E.g 6th vol Epilepsy (U.E) (p.no-145)
- In some rubrics with which condition it is associated give in brackets. E.g 6th vol (p.no 296) lower extremities
- In some rubrics for whom it is best indicated or in whom it is produced given in bracket. E.g 6th vol (p.no 296) weakness of A (in children)- carb.an
- Some rubrics are sequale of particular condition, those conditions are given in brackets. E.g 6th vol lower extremities-paralysis of legs (p.no 296)
- In some rubrics drugs are given in brackets with rubric or condition. E.g 6th vol lower extremities- patella.(p.no 297)

GRADATION
- Only one gradation. All the medicines are in roman. But few are in brackets too
- Total number of drugs – 420
- The abbreviations given for the medicines are different from other books

CHAPTERS
- Biggest chapter- Menstruation and Discharges. Total no of rubrics-1435, No of pages- 479. Vol-4
- Other big chapters are Stomach(Vol-2), Generalities and Key Notes (Vol-6), Skin (Vol-5) and eyes (Vol-1)
- Smallest chapter –Ears (59 Pages and 544 Rubrics). Vol-1
- Other small chapters are Lactation and Mammary Glands (80/622) Sleep and Dream(84/84), Bones and Limbs in General(84/541), Nose (85/650),

Hypochondria (93/435), Male Sexual Organs (99/699)
- Diagnostic and pathological rubrics are given in Generalities and keynotes chapter. E.g Anasarca, Anemia, Dropsy, Gangrene, Hypertrophy, Marasmus, Metastasis, Malignant and Typhoid
- Rubrics of mind too given in this chapter

METHOD OF SEARCHING RUBRICS
- In Searching for any desired symptom, the physician should first express it mentally or better in writing employing words commonly used and then select the word in sentence or the noun, verb or essential adjective and referring in the concordance in the responsive chapter

E.g Imagination of having two heads. Here imagination is noun as well as the central thought. The desired rubric can be found under two heading imaginations and heads

E.g Fancies seeing cats and dogs. This can be under cats, dogs and fancies of mind and disposition chapter

E.g Sensation of a stick extending from the throat to left side of abdomen, with a ball on each end of the sick. This rubric can be found under 3 headings Stick, Sensation, Abdomen of throat chapter

E.g "Sight of water causes nausea and vomiting; is not able to drink, and must close the eyes when bathing." this rubric can be found under 6 headings Sight, Water, Nausea,Vomiting, Drink, Eyes of stomach chapter

For E.g."Desires to kiss everybody"- we get that symptom as –"wants to kiss everybody. Think of the synonym "wants" or some other word in the sentence, such as "kiss" or everybody

- Frequent difficulty may be met in finding a symptom on account of difference in phraseology of the materia medica writers or upon the part of the person desiring to find the symptom. Therefore, when there is a failure to find a symptom under one word, the synonym should be thought of

For E.g: Wants to do something and yet feels no ambition While the symptom can be found referring to "do", "something" and "ambition"

- Therefore, when there is a failure to find a symptom under one word, the synonym should be thought of. For E.g: Wants to do something and yet feels no ambition

- While the symptom can be found referring to "do", " something" and "ambition" .Yet the word ' wants ' cannot be found, because the writer of the symptom did not use that word

- The word used in the materia medica is "Desires" and symptom can be found by referring to that word in the concordance

For E.g :"Desires to kiss everybody" we get that symptom as "wants to kiss everybody". Think of the synonym "wants"or some other word in the sentence, such as "kiss "or everybody"

- These volumes were not widely used. Julia M. Green characterized it was "absolutely worthless on account of bulk and repetition without useful method"

- Of the work, Kent says, "The most shameful work that ever appeared, and it is no wonder the author has gone over to Christian Science and abandoned medicine entirely. Not over 40 percent of the genuine materia medica is in this pretended complete work, while one half of Gentry's symptoms cannot be found in any materia medica. It is a mess of trash."

SPECIAL FEATURES

- Useful as a book of reference , to find the desired symptom together with the indicated remedy

- The symptoms are given in their original form (Provers own language) without much change

- In the repertory the author has used the phraseology of Materia medica without much change

- Symptoms arranged in alphabetical order under each chapter

- Symptoms can be found easily, which saves a lot of time

- One symptom can be referred to at many places

- This book could be useful for searching peculiar or a complex symptom. Which is not present in general repertoires and needs to be taken in to account for solving our problem

- If we use verb, noun or adjective of the symptom any layman can use this repertory

- Very easy to find out the rubrics as first 3 alphabets are given at the top of each page. As well as in between the rubrics (only in 1st vol)

- Few clinical hints are given after few rubrics from his clinical experience.

CRITICISM

- Majority of the rubrics consist of only one remedy. Hence cannot be used for repertorization

- Not useful for a systemic repertorization. It is only a reference book for the remedy differentiation after repertorization as the symptoms are in provers own language

- Not useful for a bedside prescription as it consists of 6 volumes

- Gradation of drugs are not given

- One who uses the book should have a thorough knowledge of synonyms

- Source of the book is not mentioned.

A COMPARATIVE STUDY OF THE TWO CONCORDANT REPERTORIES
[KNERR & GENTRY]

Differences :

	Gentry's Repertory	Knerr's Reprtory
Author	William D Gentry	C.B. Knerr
Volumes	Consists of 6 volumes	1 volume
Published in	In 1890	In 1896
Based on	The book is not based on any particular materia medica; it is collection of symptoms from all the important works at that time	Based on Hering's Guiding symptom of Materia Medica
Gradations Used	All the medicines are of four gradings used	The same grading. [I, II , I, II]
Additional Symbols	No such symbols	symbols are used in this book such as - θ, t ,π
No.of Medicines	420 medicines The number of medicines given for each symptom is less	408 medicines More number of drugs given for each symptom or rubric.
No. of Chapters	Total 30 chapters [in 6 vols]	48 chapters - from mind and disposition to drug relationship.

Similarity of the two repertories :

1. Symptoms obtained in the prover are given as such with out much alteration.

2. Alphabetical arrangement of symptoms.

CLINICAL REPERTORIES

INTRODUCTION

These sorts of repertories contain clinical symptoms/conditions with their corresponding group of medicines. They are not commonly used for the purpose of repertorization. However these repertories can be used for repertorization of cases where clinical conditions mask the characteristic symptoms of the patient. In such cases the physician finds the prominent common symptoms/clinical conditions with few modalities and concomitants. In spite of emphasis on individualized prescription based on characteristic expressions, the emergence of clinical repertories could not be prevented in homoeopathic practice even in Hahnemann's time. The grouping of the medicines according to the name of diseases, though discouraged by many stalwarts, has given birth to several clinical repertories. Master Hahnemann was certainly not happy with such kind of practice; he described it as – "Treating the names of the diseases with names of therapeutic actions".

Such a kind of practice was much favored by Dr. J Compton Burnett. He expresses it as – "The fact is, we need any and every way of finding the right remedy, the simple simile, the simple symptomatic similimum and the furthest reach of all the pathological similimum, and I maintain that we are still within the lines of Homoeopathy that is an expensive, progressive science". Dr. Burnett in his writings, has given examples of different cases i.e. like "Diseases of the Liver", "Organ diseases of Women" etc.

from where we can understand that he has preferred certain medicines for certain clinical conditions. For example- He has treated many cases of jaundice, enlargement of liver, tumor of liver by Chelidonium majus; for traumatic uterus he had used Hypericum, Arnica, Bellis per, Kali chlor, cuprum acet., Cedron etc.

Dr. J. Compton Burnett advocated more in favor of such practice but he could not compile a separate repertory for that purpose and the credit for compiling the first useful clinical repertory goes to Dr. J. H. Clarke. J. H. Clarke in the introduction of his clinical repertory has written- "Certain diseases come to have certain remedies arranged to them and all the patients who are found to be suffering from any given disease must be denoted with one of the remedies credited to it." Clinical repertory of J. H. Clarke is based on his dictionary of Materia Medica.

Though Clarke's Clinical repertory was popular at that time but O. E. Boericke's repertory gradually takes upper hand in popularity probably due to its arrangement of rubrics in different anatomical section, which is more practical and useful.

Scope and limitations of clinical repertories

Though Clinical repertories have not been put to their fullest utility, this can be very useful too if the scope and limitations are properly understood and implemented in practice.

Scope

1. Clinical repertories can be used in the study of Homoeopathic therapeutics as well as Materia Medica.

2. They help us to repertorize the following types of cases –

   a) Cases lacking in mental symptoms and physical general symptoms

   b) Cases with clinical diagnosis

   c) Cases with a few symptoms

3. They are used as quick reference books while in doubt and confusion at bedside. Not only that it also helps to reduce the number of probable medicines for a given disease condition bearing a nosological label.

4. Clinical Repertories contain some rubrics, which are not found in other general repertories; therefore they can become a good companion in the study of such rubrics.

5. Clinical repertories help us to find the most appropriate palliative medicines in incurable cases.

6. Regional repertories help in finding out the most similar medicine in a specific clinical condition.

7. In acute cases it helps best as the patient usually does not say all his symptoms during sufferings except particular symptoms.

Limitations

Clinical Repertories are based on nosological terms and clinical conditions, which are the results of clinical observations; hence their use is limited to particular type of cases. They are mainly used for reference work.

Need of pathology in prescribing

It helps to understand the symptom in context with the whole; with respect to natural history of disease and place each symptom in proper relative importance. They are important to prescribe the truly homoeopathic remedies, not the seemingly homoeopathic ones.

A. GENERAL CLINICAL REPERTORIES
I. BOERICKE'S REPERTORY

Name of the book: POCKET MANUAL OF HOMOEOPATHIC MATERIA MEDICA COMPRISING THE CHARACTERISTIC AND GUIDING SYMPTOMS OF ALL REMEDIES (CLINICAL AND PATHOGENETIC) WITH THE ADDITION OF A REPERTORY.

Author: Oscar Eugene Boericke (brother of William Boericke; a graduate from Hahnemann's Medical College; influenced very much by his brother).

Publication: The book had no repertory part in the first edition. It was added from 3rd edition onwards. The 1st Indian edition came in 1969 (*Vide ref.* It was published by Roy Publishing House, Kolkata. It contains an introduction by Dr B. K. Sarkar).

Different editions	Year of publication	Publishers	Total pgs of Pocket manual	Attached with Pocket Manual of Homoeopathic Materia Medica
1st	1906	Boericke & Runyan, New York, USA	1049	3rd edition
2nd	1912	Boericke & Tafel, Philadelphia	1155	5th edition
3rd	1916	Boericke & Runyan, New York, USA	1293	6th edition
4th	1922	Boericke & Runyan, New York,	1128	8th edition
5th	1927	Boericke & Tafel, Philadelphia USA	1042	9th edition

With the advent of the incomparable ninth edition of the progressive Pocket Manual of Homoeopathic Materia Medica, its modest companion the Repertory, has been completely remodeled and brought up to date by embodying much of the newly incorporated material. Many of the sections have been carefully rewritten and with appropriate expansion; offer a more trustworthy guide for the selection of the medicines.

Number of medicines: *1405*

Number of chapters: *25*

Construction

It has two parts. 1st part is repertory proper and 2nd part is index to repertory. Though it is called a clinical repertory it actually contains both clinical conditions and subjective symptoms i.e. appetite defective/increased/perverted; aversions/cravings. In 'Mind' chapter also we find subjective symptoms i.e. emotions, mood disposition, propensity etc.

Divisions of sections: According to Hahnemannian schema. It has 25 chapters.

1. MIND
2. HEAD
3. EYES
4. EARS
5. NOSE
6. FACE
7. MOUTH
8. TONGUE
9. TASTE
10. GUMS
11. TEETH
12. THROAT
13. STOMACH
14. ABDOMEN
15. URINARY SYSTEM
16. MALE SEXUAL SYSTEM
17. FEMALE SEXUAL SYSTEM
18. CIRCULATORY SYSTEM
19. LOCOMOTOR SYSTEM
20. RESPIRATORY SYSTEM
21. SKIN
22. FEVER
23. NERVOUS SYSTEM
24. GENERELITIES
25. MODALITIES – AGG. & AMEL.

Largest chapter – Female Sexual System

Smallest Chapter – Gums

This repertory contains almost all medicines present in the Materia Medica part by William Boericke, which has total number of 1409 medicines. The index provides a list of 1414 medicines but 5 medicines appear twice because of their dual names. For example- Cimicifuga, actea racemosa, eriodictylon, yerba santa etc.

Though this book has 1409 medicines, only 688 medicines are in narrative form. Others are given under relationship part of various medicines. Among these 688 medicines all are not described under different anatomical heads, rather only few clinical hints are given for them. Medicines under each rubric are arranged in alphabetical order in purely arbitrary and self explanatory abbreviated form. Two types of typography are used to indicate the grades of the medicines, *italics*and *roman* (italics indicate the more frequently verified clinical medicines).

Headings and subheadings: All the chapters are arranged alphabetically.

Order of headings: A specific order has been followed as mentioned below

a) *Cause: e.g.* Headache (cephalgia): Cause: bathing, bear weather changes etc.

b) *Type: e.g.* Headache (cephalgia): Type: anemic, utero-ovarian etc.

c) *Location: e.g.* Headache (cephalgia): Location: frontal, vertex etc.

d) *Character: e.g.* Headache (cephalgia): Character of pain: aching, throbbing etc.

e) *Concomitant: e.g.* Headache (cephalgia): Concomitant: anguish, yawning etc.

f) *Modalities: aggravation: e.g.* Headache (cephalgia): after drugging etc.

g) *Modalities: amelioration: e.g.* Headache (cephalgia): wrapping tightly etc.

Technical names : To emphasize the value of symptoms (more than the diagnosis) they have been bracketed e.g. **MIND** – FEAR – space (agoraphobia), EMOTIONS – Nostalgia (homesickness). But exceptions are there to this rule e.g. **MIND** – DELIRIUM – Carphologia (picking at bed clothes), **EARS** – TINNITIS AURIUM (noises in ear), **FACE** – APPEARANCE – CONDITION – Hippocratic (sickly, sunken, deathly cold).

Philosophical background: The idea of using Location, Sensation, Modality and Concomitant is similar to Bonninghausen's concept of complete symptom. The symptoms of patient are either *General* (or common symptoms) or *Peculiar* (or characteristic). The characteristic symptoms fall under:

a) Location : It shows the elective affinity of the drug. It is important because the organs are not independent instruments, but wonderfully bound together by nerves and parts most remote are in direct nerve connection.

b) Sensation or kind of action: In many drugs they are so expressive of their special action that they are expected to be present in almost in all the cases i.e. anxiety of Aconite; chilliness of Pulsatilla.

c) Modalities and concomitants: Each drug acts best under certain conditions, on certain bodily and mental constitution. Thus the most favorable ground and environment for full and free manifestation of drug individuality.

It is a fact that each symptom has Location, Sensation, Modality and Concomitant; but not possible to obtain from single or few proving (s). But the records when compiled by various provers give a complete picture. Thus, a logical breaking of symptoms and recombination later on is justifiable and verified through successes in clinical practice.

Cross references: There are three types of cross references as mentioned below-

1) To *other chapter*: after the medicines in bold letters bracketed, prefixed by 'See'. For example- NOSE – BONES – Caries: ....See Tissues (Generalities).

2) To *same chapter without medicines* i.e. for similar rubrics: prefixed by 'See'. For example- ABDOMEN – ENTERITIS – See Diarrhea.

3) To *same chapter with medicine*: after the medicines, prefixed by 'See'. These are of maximum in number. For example- URINARY SYSTEM – SEDIMENT – TYPE – cells, debris....See nephritis; FEMALE SEXUAL SYSTEM – COITION – coition, painful...See Vaginismus.

Demerits

1. Being a clinical repertory *it can never take place of a General repertory* for which the author refers to Kent, Syntheis, Knerr, Clarke etc.

2. Dr. Boericke himself says "this work found numerous suggestions based on clinical observations *or deductions from partial proving*, all of which may prove most valuable addition to our material medica, if further verified at bedside." If these suggestions had been marked, it would have enhanced the value of the book.

3. Wrong placement of certain rubrics. For example- ABDOMEN – ERUPTION – fissure, fistula, inflammation (proctitis) etc. LOCOMOTOR SYSTEM – GOUT of chest, eyes, stomach, heart etc.

4. Alphabetical arrangement is not maintained properly in whole through the repertory. For example in ABDOMEN chapter- Haemorhoids; Hernia; Intestines; Jaundice followed by Hypocondria; Liver.

5. The mistakes in printing create confusion at some places and make the search for appropriate rubric difficult. e.g.

Advantages and utility

- If characteristic symptoms are not present, it provides an easy entry point to the case.

- For therapeutic study.

- An index is provided in the repertory which makes it much useful.

- In GENERALITIES chapter- PROPHYLACTICS rubric is present which also suggest useful potencies of medicines.

- Pathology and symptoms pertaining to a part have been given together at one place, i.e.

ABDOMEN: Spleen.....; Umbilicus...; Liver-...; Diaphragm... THROAT: Pharynx...; Esophagus...; Fauces....; Uvula...

- Sensation rubric has been given as a separate rubric in STOMACH – SENSATION

- The concept of complete symptom has been incorporated in the construction of repertory. The arrangement of symptom components under various headings i.e. cause, type, location, modality etc. make it more interesting and user friendly

Highest grade single medicine rubrics

The gradation used in the repertory is based on the clinical verification of remedies. Thus it can be inferred that *single medicine rubrics found in the book should have great clinical utility.* They are given below for the purpose of clinical application by the readers:

1. Ears – auditory nerve - torpor.....*Chenop*
2. Nose – external nose - eruptions
   - scales ....*Caust*
3. Teeth - modalities - amelioration
   - hot liquids.................................*Mag. P*
4. Abdomen - cause and type
   - abuse of enema..............................*Op*
5. Female sexual system - menstruation
   - type:
   amenorrhœa - suppressed, with neuralgic
   pains about head, face.....................*Gels*
6. Female sexual system - vulva
   -labia - erysipelas, with edema.......*Apis*
7. Locomotor system - loins
   - lumbago: with sciatica..........*Rhus tox*
8. Respiratory system - voice
   - high, piping.................................*Bell*
9. Nervous system - cause -
   occurance - worse, at
   approach of thunder storm..........*Agar*

II. A CLINICAL REPERTORY TO THE DICTIONARY OF MATERIA MEDICA

Author : J.H.CLARKE

DR.CLARKE says this repertory is designed "for use in the study of the Materia Medica" and as an instrument for finding out the indicated remedies.

This repertory is compiled as an index to the dictionary of Materia Medica [3 Vol] by Clarke. This repertory will enable the practitioner to compare any remedy with any similar remedy in five different points; all of great importance in practice.

1. CLINICAL REPERTORY

2. REPERTORY OF CAUSATION

3. REPERTORY OF TEMPERAMENTS,

   ISPOSITIONS, CONSTITUTIONS, AND STATES

4. REPERTORY TO THE CLINICAL RELATIONSHIPS

5. REPERTORY TO THE NATURAL RELATIONSHIP

PART - I CLINICAL REPERTORY

The clinical repertory presented here with constitutes the index to the heading of "clinical" in the dictionary of practical Materia Medica. In the dictionary every drug is described from a number of different point of view. The clinical point of view is one of these, and under the heading clinical Clarke has prefixed to each remedy a list of the affections in which it has been found most frequently indicated in practice. In compiling these clinical lists Clarke had in view the project of preparing, later on, an index of these headings.

Unlike in the dictionary and prescriber the names of the remedies are italicized in the clinical repertory in front of a clinical rubric. The drugs which are given in italics shows that these drugs are also given in the prescribe and dictionary and those which appear in ordinary print are the drugs which are added afterwards by the author.

The chief problem of scientific therapeutics consists in the discovering of indications for remedies. All ways of finding indications are open to practitioner and the clinical avenue is one of them. In Homoeopathy any remedy may be required in any case of any disease. The occurrence of the name of any remedy under the heading of any disease shows that in its action it has a general correspondence with the most marked feature of cases of that disease.

It will frequently happen that the practitioner will have in mind a number of remedies which more or less closely correspond to a given case, and when he consults the clinical repertory this knowledge will enable him at once to pick out of the list there presented the most similar remedy to his case. If still any doubt the prescriber has to consult dictionary, in which each of the remedies named in the repertory will be bound described individually in detail.

The use of the nosological correspondence is one method by means of which a similar, if not the most similar remedy may be discovered. Another method is by ascertaining the similarity of specificity of seat. Some drugs have a predominant affinity for certain organs, and these drugs will often relieve a great variety of affections seated in, or arising from diseases of these particular organs. In compiling clinical repertory many general heading such as "liver diseases of ", spleen affection of, are given. The lists of remedies given under these headings will show the drugs, which have been observed to hit these organs hardest, and will there by give a very important point for comparison.

While the compilation of this work was in progress Dr.Clarke thought that it would greatly extend the usefulness of the clinical repertory if he were to add one or two other indications at the same time. So he compiled indices under other headings like causation, temperament, and relationship of remedies.

CLINICAL RUBRICS FOUND IN PART- I ARE:

1. Acetonaemia
2. Acidity.
3. Acne
4. Acromegaly
5. Addison's disease.
6. Adrenal neuralgia.
7. Adrenal neuralgia.
8. Alopecia.
9. Anaemia.
10. Beriberi
11. Biliary colic
12. Blepharitis
13. Brachial neuralgia
14. Brights disease.
15. Burns
16. Bursitis
17. Calculus
18. Cellulitis
19. Chalazion
20. Cheloid
21. Chickenpox
22. Ciliary neuralgia
23. Coccygodynia
24. Cold abscess
25. Decubitus
26. Dengue fever
27. Diabetes
28. Diptheria
29. Dissect wounds
30. Dupuytrens contracture
31. Dysmenorrhoea
32. Dyspepsia
33. Eclampsia
34. Ecchymosis
35. Eczema
36. Elephantiasis
37. Embolus
38. Emphysema
39. Empyema
40. Entericfever
41. Fatty degeneration
42. Fatty tumour
43. Fibroma
44. Fissures
45. Fistula
46. Freckles
47. Gallstones
48. Ganglion
49. Gangrene

50. Gastritis
51. German measles
52. Glaucoma
53. GOITRE
54. Gout
55. Hematocoele
56. Hayfever
57. Hemiplegia
58. Herpes
59. Hodgkins disease
60. Hydrocoele
61. Hypopyon
62. Impetigo
63. Impotence
64. JAUNDICE
65. Keratitis
66. Knock knee
67. Landrys paralysis
68. Laryngitis
69. Lead colic
70. Lipoma
71. Malaria
72. Marasmus
73. Mastitis
74. Measles
75. Meniers disease
76. Migraine
77. Morvans dis
78. Mumps
79. Myopia
80. Myxdeama
81. Naevus
82. Nasal polyps
83. Necrosis
84. Night blindness

85. Optic neuritis
86. Orchitis
87. Osteomylitis
88. Osteoma
89. Pancreatitis
90. Paralysis agitans
91. Parotitis
92. Pellagra
93. Pemphigus
94. Pernicious anaemia
95. Phlebitis
96. Plague
97. Pleurisy
98. Pneumonia
99. Potts disease
100. Psoriasis
101. Rabies
102. Raynaud's disease
103. Renal calculi
104. Rheumatoid arthritis
105. Rickets
106. Riggs disease
107. Scabies
108. Sciatica
109. Scurvy
110. Smallpox
111. Sterility
112. Stomatitis
113. Sycosis
114. Syphilis
115. Syringomyelia
116. Tabes mesentrica
117. Thrombosis
118. Tic dourolx
119. Tonsillitis

120. Trifacial nerve paralysis

121. Tuberculosis

122. Typhoid fever

123. Typhus fever

124. Leukaemia

125. Cellulitis

126. Urticaria

127. Varicella

128. Varicocoele

129. Varicose vein

130. Warts

131. Uraemia

132. Urethritis

133. Wens

134. whooping cough

135. writers cramps

136. Xerostoma

137. Yellow fever

138. Zoster

PART II - REPERTORY OF CAUSATION

DR. CLARKE has described in his dictionary the remedies under the heading causation. This tells how remedies are related to conditions due to definite causes. Therefore he has added an alphabetical list of causes, under any one of which will be bound named all the drugs, which have been observed to be curative in conditions produced by it.

Almost all remedies have relations of some kind to the various accidents and conditions of ordinary life. Their symptoms are made worse or better by heat or cold, rest or motion, by night or by day or other circumstances or conditions. Many remedies are related to the effects of certain conditions. Although causation and

aggravation are not the same, they are closely allied. Thus is related to the effects of damp weather, and appears in the list of remedies having this causation; but it also has its symptoms, when not caused by damp, aggravated in a supreme degree by conditions of damp. Therefore the prescriber who uses this list of causes as a rough list of aggravations also will not go wrong.

The names of a few remedies have been added which do not occur in the dictionary of Materia Medica. They are given in brackets. When a cause is associated with any particular effect, that effect is placed in brackets and precedes the name of the remedy, which corresponds to it. For ex - "washing clothes" causes ill effects to which certain remedies correspond. Phosphorous corresponds to headache resulting from washing clothes. In the list of remedies this fact is marked thus "headache - phos". When in a list of remedies, one of them has a qualifying word or phrase thus prefixed to it, the qualification must be understood to apply to that remedy only, and not to those which follow.

RUBRICS. FOUND IN THIS PART ARE:

1. Acid food

2. Alcoholism

3. Arms, raising.

4. Anger.

5. Bathing.

6. Business embarrassment

7. Bread.

8. Butter.

9. Cabbage

10. Carrying heavy wt.

11. Checked eruptions.

12. Cheese.	46. Indigestible food.
13. Chill.	47. Injured pride.
14. Climbing mountains.	48. Injuries to nerve.
15. Coffee	49. Influenza.
16. Contradiction effects of	50. Jarring.
17. Coryza	51. Jealousy.
18. Damp	52. Journeys, long.
19. Dentition.	53. Joy, sudden.
20. Discharges suppressed.	54. Labour, mental.
21. Disappointments.	55. Laughing.
22. Dog bites.	56. Lead.
23. Draft of air.	57. Lemonade.
24. Dry cold winds.	58. Light, bright.
25. Early rising.	59. Lifting.
26. Eggs, bad.	60. Lochia, suppressed.
27. Emotional disturbance.	61. Mechanical injuries.
28. Examination	62. Melons.
29. Exertion,	63. Menses, suppressed.
- Bodily	64. Mental, excitement / application.
- Mental.	65. Mercury.
30. Eyes, injuries to.	66. Milk.
31. Fasting.	67. Music.
32. Feet, wetting.	68. News, bad.
33. Fevers.	69. Nettle rash, suppressed.
34. Flowers (fainting)	70. Night watching.
35. Fright.	71. Noise.
36. Fruit.	72. Odor strong.
37. Gas light.	73. Onions.
38. Gonorrhoea.	74. Operation.
39. Grief.	75. Opium.
40. Haemorrhages.	76. Otorrhoea, suppressed.
41. Hair cutting.	77. Over eating.
42. Head blow on.	78. Over exertion.
43. Hot weather.	79. Over strain.
44. Ice cream.	80. Over study.
45. Ice water.	81. Pain.

82. Passion, fit of.
83. Pastry
84. Perspiration checked.
85. Pork.
86. Pregnancy.
87. Ptomaine poisoning.
88. Punctured wounds.
89. Quinine.
90. Rage.
91. Rains, drenching.
92. Rice.
93. Rich food.
94. Riding in carriage.
95. Salt.
96. Salty food.
97. Skin affections checked.
98. Shock.
99. Sleep loss of.
100. Ship, riding in a.
101. Snowy air.
102. Spinal injuries, old.
103. Sprains.
104. Stone cutting.
105. Strains.
106. Strong odors.
107. Sugar.
108. Summer.
109. Sun.
110. Suppressed anger.
111. Surgical operations.
112. Sweat suppression of.
113. Tea.
114. Temperature change of.
115. Thunder.
116. Tight boots.
117. Tobacco.
118. Traveling.
119. Typhoid fever.
120. Unpleasant news.
121. Unripe fruit.
122. Unusual excitement.
123. Vaccination.
124. Vegetables
125. Venesection.
126. Wading.
127. Walking.
128. Washing.
129. Water.
130. Weather.
131. Winds.
132. Wines.
133. Winter.
134. Worry.
135. Wounds.
136. Yawning.

PART III - REPERTORY OF TEMPERAMENTS, DISPOSITIONS, CONSTITUTIONS, AND STATES

In this list are given the remedies, which have been found to act most beneficially in certain types of persons, temperaments, sex and age. There are also included complaints and conditions of particular types of persons and constitutions. In the dictionary of Materia Medica these are generally given in the section characteristics under the description "suited to".

Acute observers, from the time of Hahnemann onwards, have noticed that some remedies act well on some types of persons and not at all so well on other. The respective types of nux vomica and pulsatilla are well known; but many other remedies have preferences more or less well marked for particular temperaments.

This index is very important because the type of constitution is very often determining factor in the choice of a remedy. There are some patients whose constitution correspond so accurately to a particular medicinal type, that the corresponding remedy will cure almost any indisposition they may happen to have. So this sect6ion becomes a complement of the clinical repertory. The user of this repertory, therefore, who may not find the remedy he is in search of in the clinical repertory, may possibly find it in the repertory of temperaments, under the heading of the complaint the patient is suffering from.

CONSTITUTIONS:

1. Asthmatic.
2. Bilious.
3. Broken down.
4. Carbo nitrogenoid.
5. Debilitated.
6. Delicate.
7. Dry.
8. Feeble.
9. Gouty.
10. Hydrogenoid.
11. Lax, fibre with.
12. Leucophlegmatic.
13. Nervo-sanguine / sanguinine.
14. Nervous.
15. Neuralgic.
16. Phthisical.
17. Psoric.
18. Scorbutic.
19. Scrofulous.
20. Slow, torpid.
21. Weakly.

DISPOSITIONS:

1. Affectionate.
2. Gay.
3. Gentle.
4. Hasty.
5. Haughty.
6. Haughty, when sick.
7. Irritable.
8. Malicious.
9. Melancholic.
10. Mild.
11. Sad.
12. Spiteful, malicious.
13. Tenacious & Irrascible.
14. Voluptous.
15. Yielding.

TEMPERAMENTS:

1. Bilious.
2. Brunette.
3. Choleric.
4. Excitable.
5. Hasty.
6. Hysterical.
7. Impatient.
8. Indolent.
9. Irresolute.
10. Irritable.
11. Lax,
12. Leucophlegmatic.
13. Lymphatic.
14. Lyphatic - Nervous.
15. Melancholic.
16. Mild.
17. Mischievous.
18. Nervous.

19. Phlegmatic.
20. Restless.
21. Sanguine.
22. Sensitive.
23. Slow, torpid.

OTHER RUBRICS FOUND UNDER PART- III

1. Accomplishes little though busy all the time.
2. Acidity, colic or spasms with, of infants.
3. Aged persons.
4. Agitation, nervous.
5. Alcoholism, chronic insomnia of.
6. Anaemia.
7. Animal heat diminished, constitutions with.
8. Assimilating power lack of.
9. Babies, colic of.
10. Big bellied children.
11. Body has a filthy smell, not removed by washing.
12. Breathlessness & fatigue, with flushed cheeks.
13. Bronchitis in old persons.
14. Cancers & glandular enlargements.
15. Catarrh, disposed to.
16. Chalky look, persons of.
17. Children:
    - Abdomen, large with.
    - Big bellied
    - Big heads with
    - Chubby, fat
    - Clumsy
    - Convulsions of
    - Cross, outrageously
    - Dainty & capricious

- Delicate, sickly
- Emaciated
- Excitable
- Fair
- Fat & bloated

18. Damp, cold changes persons who take cold from.
19. Debility, nervous after influenza.
20. Defective nutrition.
21. Despair of perfect recovery.
22. Destructive tendency, persons of.
23. Diarrhoea:
    - Chronic sufferers, from
    - Early, stages of
    - Profuse, watery, of old people
24. Diathesis:
    - Gouty
    - Lithic or sycotic
    - Psoric
    - Rheumatic
    - Scrofulous
    - Scrofulous or Mercurial
25. Elderly persons.
26. Emaciated children.
27. Exhausted by disease.
28. Exercise, mental / physical, aversion to.
29. Extremities, cold, sallow people with.
30. Fasting, persons who have bowel complaints from.
31. Fear, terror & timidity.
32. Feeble, digestive powers.
33. Feet, soles of, hot.
34. Glands affections of, Persons having.
35. Gouty complaints.
36. Growth children of, irregular.
37. Haemorrhagic patients

38. Hands, fetid sweat on.
39. Imbecility.
40. Indolent persons.
41. Infancy, complaints during.
42. Jealous.
43. Jovial.
44. Jaundiced complexion.
45. Keen intellect with feeble muscular development.
46. Lack of animal heat.
47. Lack of reaction.
48. Lean persons.
49. Marasmus, children with.
50. Memory weak, persons of.
51. Milk, children who cannot take.
52. Neuritis, traumatic.
53. Nose-bleed of children.
54. Newborn children.
55. Obesity.
56. Old age.
57. Old looking children.
58. Pale children.
59. Pallor, lips of.
60. Perception quick.
61. Quick tempered persons.
62. Quinine, cases previously maltreated with.
63. Rapid progress of disease.
64. Red face.
65. Relaxed fibre.
66. Sallow people with cold extremities.
67. Scorbutic conditions.
68. Sedentary habits, persons of.
69. Tea drinkers, colic of.
70. Teething children.
71. Timid persons.

72. Tired feeling extending into limbs.
73. Ulcers, deep, thin patients with.
74. Urine, red sediment in.
75. Uterine disorders.
76. Vaccination, ailments from.
77. Venous constitution with tendency to haemorrhoids.
78. Warts on the palms.
79. Weak children.
80. Weakened by long sickness.
81. Wrinkled skin.
82. Yawning, complaints which are concomitant to.
83. Yellow skin.
84. Yellow saddle across nose, pot bellied mothers with.

PART IV REPERTORY TO THE CLINICAL RELATIONSHIPS

This section of the repertory gives in tabular form the chief clinical relations of all remedies of the Materia Medica so far as they have been noted. They are included under the following heading:

1. Complementary remedies
2. Remedy follows well
3. Remedy is followed well by
4. Compatible remedies
5. Incompatible remedies
6. Remedy antidotes
7. Remedy is antidoted by
8. Duration of action

The term compatible is generic term and includes all the remedies of the first three columns. Some remedies have been observed to prepare the way for other remedies; some to follow other well such remedies are termed compatible remedies.

Some spoil the effects of other, and such are called incompatibles.

When a remedy has done well and has ceased to be indicated, the choice of the remedy to follow will be greatly assisted by knowledge of clinical relationships. In comparing the table Dr. Clarke has made use of the excellent table published by Dr. Gibson Miller.

PART V - REPERTORY OF NATURAL RELATIONSHIP

The homoeopathic Materia Medica consists potentially we may say, of anything and everything that may be found in the universe. Man himself epitomises the universe, and nothing in the universe can therefore be said to be unrelated to him.

The repertory of natural relationships shows at a glance the place in nature of any remedy in question mineral, vegetable or animal and how it stands in regards to its closest congeners. In the dictionary is given the natural order of each plant. In the repertory will be found an alphabetical list of all the natural orders represented, and under each is given In alphabetical order a list of all the plants of that order included in the Materia Medica.

But there is also given a list of the natural orders in their systematic or evolutionary order; so that very order is here given in juxtra position with its allied orders. In this list a number is prefixed to each order; and in the alphabetical list is given each order the same number.

The following list shows remedies belonging to different kingdoms of nature arranged in order of their natural kinship. The list will enable readers to find how almost any given remedy in Materia medica

is related to any other remedy in nature. The list comprise:

1. **Metals or elements.**
2. **The Vegetable kingdom.**
3. **The Animal kingdom.**
4. **Sarcodes.**
5. **Nosodes.**

1. Metals or elements

An alphabetical list of the elements represented is given, each with its symbol & atomic weight. Prefixed to each name is a number. This number shows its position in the succeeding list, which gives the elements in the order of their atomic weights. In addition to this distinguishing number in the second list is affixed the letter "G " & a Roman numeral. This refers to a third list - a list of the Mendeleeffian Groups; & the numeral shows in which of these groups any given element is to be found. E.g.

Alphabetical list

- 10. Aluminium ....Al 27.10
- 44. Aurum.................Au 197.20
- 48. Bismuthum............Bi 208.50
- 28. Bromium...............Br 79.96
- 33. (Cadmium) ....Cd 112.40
- 16. (Calcium) ....Ca 40.10 etc.

Note: The numerals prefixed to the names in this list show the place of each element in the list following, arranged in the order of the atomic weights.

The brackets signify that the element named is represented in the materia medica only by its salts.

List in order of Atomic weights

1. G I - Hydrogenium – – 1.008
2. G I - Lithium – – – – – – – 7.03
3. G III - Boron – – – – – – – 11.00

4. G IV - Carbon ― ― ― ― ― 12.00
5. G V - Nitrogenium ― ― 14.04
6. G VI - Oxygenium ― ― 16.00
7. G VII - Flurinum ― ― ― ― 19.00 etc.

Note: The letters " G I" refers to the list following & show the group of elements to which the particular element belongs.

Groups according to Mendeleeff (Group I - Group VIII)

- Group I
  o Lithium
  o A.
    - Natrum
    - Kali
  o B.
    - Hydrogenium
    - Cuprum
    - Argentum
    - Aurum
- Group II
  o A.
    - Magnesium
    - Calcium
    - Strontium
    - Barium
  o B.
    - Zincum
    - Cadmium
    - Mercurius
- etc. till Group VIII

2. VEGETABLE KINGDOM

There are two lists given in this section - a list of natural orders in alphabetical order & a list of natural orders in systematic or evolutionary order. In the first or alphabetical list, under the name of each order, all the remedies of the order are given, also alphabetically. The alphabetical list is distinguished by numbers which correspond with the numbers of the systematic list, so that the place of any remedy in each list can at once be found. E.g.

Natural Botanical Orders

1) Alphabetical list of natural botanical orders represented in materia medica
- Algae (119)
- Fucus vesiculosus
- Amaryllidaceae (101)
- Agave Americana
- Narcissus
- Anacardiaceae
- Anacardium Occidentale
- Anacardium Orientale
- Comocladia
- Rhus Aromatica
- Rhus Diversiloba
- Rhus Glabra
- Rhus radicans
- Rhus Toxicodendron
- Rhus venenata
- Schinus
- Berberidaceae (5)
- Berberis aquifolium
- Berberis vulgaris.
- Caulophyllum
- Podophyllum
- Cistaceae (11)
- Cistus Canadensis
- Droseraceae (38)
- Drosera.
- etc.

Note: The number affixed to each natural order shows the place of the order in the systematic arrangement given in the succeeding section.

2) List of natural Botanical orders represented in the materia medica in systematic arrangement.

Division 1 - **Phanerogamia** → Sub-Division 1 - **Angiospermia** → Class 1 - **Dicotyledones** → Sub-class 1 - **Polypetalae** →

> Series 1 - Thalamiflorae
1. (1) Ranunculaceae
2. (2) Magnoliaceae
3. (3) Anonaceae
4. (4) Menispermaceae
5. (5) Berberidaceae
6. (6) Nymphaeaceae
7. Etc. till (19)

> Series 2 - Disciflorae
1. (20) Linaceae
2. (21) Zygophyllaceae
3. (22) Geraniaceae
4. etc. till (32)

> Series 3 - Calyciflorae
1. (34) Leguminosae
    o Papilionaceae
    o Mimoseae
2. (35) Rosaceae
    o Drupaceae
    o Pomeae
    o Roseae
3. (36) Saxifragaceae
4. etc. till (50)

→ Sub class 2 - **Gamopetalae (or Corolliflorae)**
> Series 1 - Inferoe (or Epigynoe)
1. (51) Caprifoliaceae
2. (52) Rubiaceae
3. (53) Valerianaceae
4. etc. till (55)

> Series 2 - Superae (or Heteromerae)
1. (56) Ericaceae
2. (57) Plumbaginaceae
3. (58) Primulaceae

> Series 3 - Dicarpiae
1. (60) Oleaceae
2. (61) Jasminaceae
3. (62) Apocynaceae
4. etc. till (75)

→ Sub class 3 - **Monochlamydeae (or incompleteae)**
> Series 1 - Curvembryeae
1. (76) Chenopodiaceae
2. (77) Phytolaccaceae
3. (78) Polygonaceae
4. etc. till (95)

→ Class 2 - **Monocotyledones**
1. (96) Orchidaceae
2. (97) Zingiberaceae
3. (98) Musaceae
4. etc. till (102)

→ Division- 2
1. (103) Liliaceae
2. (104) Smilaceae
3. (105) Melanthaceae
4. etc. till (113)

→ Sub division 2 - **Gymnospermia**
1. (114) Coniferae
2. (115) Gnetaceae

→ Division 2 - **Cryptogamia**
1. (116) Equisetaceae
2. (117) Filices
3. (118) Lycopodiaceae

3. ANIMAL KINGDOM

Of the animal kingdom a similar arrangement has been adopted - an alphabetical list distinguished by numbers corresponding to numbers in the succeeding systematic list.

1. Alphabetical list of natural orders
   1. Acaridea (16)
   2. Trombidium
   3. Bufonidae (25)
   4. Bufo
   5. Carnivora (31)
   6. Mephitis
   7. Diptera (7)
   8. Culex musca
   9. Erytherineae (22)
   10. Erythrimus
   11. Fibrospongiae (91)
   12. Badiaga
   13. Spongia
   14. Gorgoniaeceae (3)
   15. Corallium Rubrum
   16. Helodermidae (30)
   17. Heloderma
   18. Isopoda (13)
   19. Oniscus
   20. etc.

2. Natural Zoological orders in systematic arrangement.

4. **Sarcodes:** These are prepared from healthy animal tissues and secretions

5. **Nosodes:** These are prepared from morbid animal tissues and secretions

Special Features:

1) The rubrics like babies, children, constitution, Girls, hysterical, infants, old age, women are well presented .

2) No gradation of drugs given.

3) This repertory has 1063 medicines, but 52 abbreviations have appeared twice hence the actual number of medicines in this repertory has 1011.

I. BELLS DIARRHOEA

Repertory:- "THE HOMOEPATHIC THERAPEUTICS OF DIARRHOEA, DYSENTERY, CHOLERA MORBUS, CHOLERA INFANTUM, AND ALL OTHER LOOSE EVACUATIONS OF THE BOWELS"

Author: **Dr. James B. Bell**

INTRODUCTION

Homoeopathy was born in 1796 and in spite of its spread and propagation all over the world with innumerable remarkable cures, we have to fight for its recognition and prove its scientificity. In 19th century and later part of 20th century, homoeopathy has proved its worth by checking, curing and preventing many of the epidemics of various fatal diseases. At one time cholera was one of such dreaded diseases. Hahnemann and later his disciples have been repeatedly successful to cure cholera and other diarrheal diseases. Diarrhea, cholera, dysentery and other such conditions of the bowels is one of the most common complain we encounter in our daily practice and sometimes most difficult to treat. Moreover the failure to treat such cases was not considered the failure of the physician but of the whole system. It was the difficulty of treating these that first awakened the desire to possess in one little work all that was known of our Materia Medica as applied to disturbed evacuations of the bowels. Hence emerged the work is as "THE HOMOEPATHIC THERAPEUTICS OF DIARRHOEA, DYSENTERY, CHOLERA MORBUS, CHOLERA INFANTUM, AND ALL OTHER LOOSE EVACUATIONS OF THE BOWELS" by Dr. James B. Bell.

THE AUTHOR

James Bachelder Bell (1859- 1914) – Not much detail is known about James Bachelder Bell. He was born in the year 1838. He graduated from Homoeopathic Medical College of Philadelphia in 1859. He was the president of the International Hahnemannian Association in 1892. And he died in the year 1914.

THE BOOK

According to the classification of repertories it is designated as a type of special clinical repertory.

Plan and construction: Following the traditional repertories, this book consists of 2 sections viz- therapeutics and repertory. This kind of typical arrangement by the Master multiplies the function of books. It is meant for study of Materia Medica and to be utilized at the bed-side at the same time.

Part I – The Remedies and their Indications

Part II – Repertory

Part I contains the remedies and their indications. Each remedy is described under the following heads-

- Stool
- Aggravation
- Amelioration
- Before stool
- During stool
- After stool
- Accompaniments

The last paragraph under each medicine contains valuable information which is of immense clinical importance.

Part II contains the Repertory, which has the following sections:

1. Pathological names

2. Character of the stools

3. Condition of the stools and of the accompanying symptoms

    i. Aggravations; ii. Ameliorations

4. Accompaniments of the Evacuations

    i. Before stool; ii. During stool; iii. After stool

5. General Accompaniments

a) Mind and Mood
b) Head
c) Eyes and ears
d) Nose
e) Face
f) Mouth
g) Throat
h) Oesophagus
i) Appetite
j) Eructation
k) Nausea and Vomiting
l) Stomach
m) Abdomen
n) Anus
o) Urine
p) Sexual organs
q) Chest
r) Back and neck
s) Extremities
t) Sleep
u) Fever
    – Chill
    – Heat
    – Sweat
    – Pulse
v) Skin
w) General symptoms

YEAR OF PUBLICATION

- 1ST EDITION- 1869
- 2ND EDITION- 1881
- 3RD EDITION- 1888
- 4TH EDITION- 1896
- 11TH EDITION- 1920

This book has undergone fifteen editions till now.

CLASSIFICATION OF MEDICINES

This is talked about in 2nd edition by Dr. W.T. Liard and is divided into four classes-

- 1st – remedies which have been thoroughly proved and repeatedly verified in practice
- 2nd – remedies which have also been well proved, but whose symptoms, as yet, lack clinical information
- 3rd – medicines which possess only fragmentary and imperfect pathogeneses. These may be styled "the suggestive remedies" and include such drugs as *Coto Bark, Gent. Lut., Geran., Hura., Oenothera, Paullinia*, etc.
- 4th–remedies whose indications are derived solely *ab us in morbis*

CHARACTER OF THE WORK

This work is intended to apply to all loose evacuations of the bowels, and to describe them, their aggravations and ameliorations, with their immediate accompaniments and general accompanying symptoms.

The 1st heading comes as 'Stool' under which different character of the stool has been described.

Under the head of 'Aggravations' and 'Ameliorations' those influences are given which affect the stool, and also those which act as excited causes of the attack. When referring to other symptoms, they will be found indicated in parentheses. The concomitants of the stool like 'before stool', 'during stool' and 'after stool' have been described thereafter. Then it follows the general accompaniments, which include all the symptoms that can occur during the attack.

Under each of the best known remedies some symptoms are found italicized. These are the symptoms which have been most frequently observed, and which also serve to most sharply distinguish that remedy from others. While there are some symptoms which are especially characteristic; they are printed in **black type**.

It is intended to include not just every remedy that has been known to purge, but only every remedy of which enough is known, either of its stools, or conditions, or concomitants, to distinguish it from any other remedy.

TYPOGRAPHY : The remedies are seen in four typographies-

Bold Roman
- *Italic*
- Roman
- (Roman): The medicines written in bracket are doubtful remedies.

Though it is not very clear as to what typography represents which grade but it may be considered that the four classes described in the preface to 2nd edition correspond to these typographies.

NO. OF MEDICINES
141 medicines are used in the therapeutic section.

In 2nd edition 32 remedies were added. In 3rd edition 4 remedies of little importance have been omitted viz.: Cactus, Euphorb., Opuntia and Castoreum. 5 medicines considered to be of much value have been added, viz.: Acetic ac., Crotalus, Angustura, Carbolic ac. and Valeriana. In 4th edition no addition or deletion of drugs is done.

PURPOSE OF THIS BOOK
- For author's own use as a labor-saver
- As a receptacle for clinical observations
- For gleanings from others and from the periodicals

ABOUT SELECTION OF REMEDY
The selection of remedy is done by seeking the remedy which possesses the physical and diagnostic symptoms of the case, and which corresponds also to the special, distinguishing and peculiar symptoms which mark the individual case. And further, if a remedy is found that possesses distinctly the latter symptoms, but not, so far as is known, the former, we may conclude safely that it does possess the former, and administer it with confidence.

ABOUT THE POTENCY SELECTION
One of the shortcomings of repertories is that they are silent regarding the potency selection. That has been overcome by use of the 12th, 15th, 30th, 200th, and often higher potencies, of our remedies, administered in water, and repeated every 1-6 hours

according to the urgency of the symptoms, and suspended as soon as decided improvement appeared. If the same remedy was needed to be resumed again, it has seemed to do better in a higher potency, but on this point we cannot yet speak with entire assurance.

SOME RUBRICS FROM REPERTORY

Character of stool

1. Colourless, increasingly and watery- Coloc.

2. Expulsion, sputtering, spattering all over the vessel- Natr. S.

3. Fecal, black and hard, first part, last part white as milk- Aescul.

4. Infrequent, long intervals between- Arn.

5. Soap-suds like- *Benz. Ac.*

6. Tomato sauce like- Apis

7. Undigested, food of previous day- **Oleand**.

8. White, shining particles like kernels of rice- *Cub.*

9. Whey-like- *Iod.*

Condition of the stool and of the accompanying symptoms

Aggravation

1. Acute diseases after- *Carbo v, China., Psor.*

2. Alone, when- *Stram.*

3. Chocolate, after- Bor. *Lith c.*

4. Cold, becoming when- *Coccul.*

5. Drastic medicines after- *Nux v.*

6. Drinks, alcoholic after- Lach.

7. Meat, fresh- *Caust.*

8. Nephritis during- *tereb.*

9. News, bad- **Gels**

Amelioration

1. Drinks cold- **Phos**

2. Drinks hot- Chel.

3. Milk, hot- Croton tig.

4. Smoking- Coloc.

Accompaniments of the evacuations

Before stool

1. Ill humour- bor., *Calc. c*

2. Mucous, white discharge of- Kali c.

3. *Ptyalism-* Fluor. Ac.

During stool

1. Back, chill in- *Thromb.*

2. Head, fore, cold sweat on- *Verat.*

3. Head, fore, warm sweat on- *Merc.v.*

4. Hunger- *Aloe*

5. Uterus, bearing down pain in- Bell

After stool

1. Chilliness- *canth.,* Grat., Mez.

2. Hunger, canine- Lept., *Petrol.*

3. Irritation, ill humour- Nitr.ac.

4. Sleep as soon as tenesmus ceases- Colch., Sulp.

5. Water brash- *Caust.*

COMPONENTS OF A TOTALITY

1. Pathological type is considered whether the symptoms correspond to diarrhea, dysentery or cholera.

2. Character of stool regarding colour, smell, consistency etc. is to be taken.

3. Modalities include ailments from, aggravation and ameliorations.

4. Accompanying symptoms before, during and after stool is considered.

5. General accompaniments which are actually the symptoms of the patient help for the final differentiation between the close running remedies.

UTILITY

- This repertory is a complete work as it has expressed not only the symptoms of the bowel but the general state of the patient too. The section on General Accompaniments justifies this.

- Accompanying symptoms before, during and after is well elaborated in separate sub-sections.

- Handy and easy for reference as the sections in the repertory can be referred quickly and the medicine can be selected accurately without much hassle.

- *Desires and Aversions* related to food items are mentioned in **Appetite** sub-section.

- This book also mentions the guidelines regarding the selection of the remedy and also its potency selection.

LIMITATIONS

- Number of remedies mentioned is less in this repertory. As the author has included only those remedies of which enough is known either in its stool, or conditions or concomitants to distinguish it from any other remedy.

Moreover the author has not included medicines-

- Whose proving is indefinite. This the author has said in context to a much larger number of medicines given in Allen's Symptom Register (425) and Kneer's Repertory of the Guiding Symptoms (159)

- Where diarrhea is simply accessory to a larger and more important group of symptoms E.g. *Diadema* in Intermittent fever, *Asterias rubens* in Epilepsy or *Arum triphyllum* in Typhoid or Scarlet fever and not well defined in itself.

- While describing under the heading 'Character of the stools' many sub rubrics are found which do not actually correspond with the meaning of the main rubric. E.g. Involuntary, Expulsion difficult, Alternating with constipation.

CONCLUSION

Though clinical repertories have not been put to their fullest utility, these can be very useful too if the scope and limitations are properly understood and implemented in practice. But while going through this special clinical repertory and its construction we see that the author has well justified its utility and at the same time not compromised with the Hahnemannian principle of totality and individualization. T.F. Allen says "A good clinical repertory is certainly a desideratum that is something always wanted and needed"

II. BERRIDGES EYE REPERTORY

INTRODUCTION : Complete Repertory to the Homoeopathic Materia Medica on diseases of the eye (commonly known as Berridge's Repertory of Eye) is authored by Dr. E. W. Berridge in April 1873. The main source for the book was C.Hering's Materia Medica and addition from later provings but Berridge also added many valuable symptoms from cases of poisoning, reported in the allopathic journals.

Dr. C. Hering commented about the book as

"it is the only complete one we have , it is the clearest and best arranged and it will enable us to do twice as much as formerly in diseases of the eyes"

Plan and Construction :

The Repertory is constructed in such a form that Each chapter of is divided into two sections:

Section-I: the symptoms themselves.

It is further divided into 5 subsections

I A - functional symptoms

I B - Anatomical regions

I C - General character, sequence & directions

I D - Right side

I E - Left side.

Section – II : their conditions (including concomitants)

It is further divided into 2 subsections.

II A – aggravations

II B – Ameliorations

The conditions including the concomitant are arranged in 23 groups as follows:

1] Time,

2] Situation and external influences,

3] Posture,

4] Touch,

5] Motion

6] Head (including mental symptoms),

7] Eyes.

8] Ears,

9] Nose,

10] Face and front of neck,

11] Teeth,

12] Mouth and throat,

13] Abdomen (including stomach, anus and all functional symptoms there of,

14] Urinary organs,

15] Sexual organs

16] Chest and larynx,

17] Back and nape of neck,

18] Arms,

19] Legs,

20] Sleep,

21] Fever (chills, heat, sweat),

22] Generalities (including skin, Bones, convulsions, other drugs etc).

All the symptoms in these subsections are arranged alphabetically, excepting the peculiar symptoms, which not falling under any general heading are placed last. All symptoms of a nearly identical meaning are placed under the same rubric, according to the table of synonyms. The arrangement of the symptoms in section –II is in every respect exactly the same as that of section I.

In the subsection I C direction, the

symptoms are given in the chapter belonging to the organ in which they commence, thus "shooting from eyeball to head" is given in the subsection I C of the chapter on "eyes", but not in that on "Head".

Sometimes in a complex group of symptoms one symptoms follows another; in this case if they are both in the same organ they are given in section I. Subsection C; if in different organs, in section II. Thus " Blindness followed by heat in eyes" would be given in IC. Under the rubric " symptoms changing character", but "Blindness followed by heat in head" would be given in II under rubric " Before head symptoms", and also in the head chapter under "after eye symptoms".

Collectives of medicines agreeing with regard to anatomical regions, the chief divisions of the functional symptoms, general character, sequence, direction, and sides, are given under their respective rubrics, and in these collectives doubtful symptoms only are bracketed. In these collectives also, the principle one contains the less; thus under the general rubric "Eye to face" are given all the medicines which have any variety of the above e.g., "Eye to lower jaw", to make the collective complete; but, "shooting from eyeball to lower jaw" is given under the latter rubric only, and not under both.

In the rubrics "right then left", "above then below", and the reverse, clinical symptoms are marked with an asterisk, to facilitate the application of Hering's low of inverse directions.

In the last the General chapter, the arrangement is similar to that of the preceding ones. First is the arrangement according to specific character, the medicines to which belong any variety of symptom (e.g. shooting) in any part of the body being arranged under their respective rubrics, next comes the arrangements according to tissues (e.g., glands, skin, bones, entire body etc.) which correspond to the Anatomical regions of the preceding chapter; followed by general character sequence and direction, right side and left side, just as before. In the conditions of this chapter the same rule is observed; thus under aggravation " by warmth" we have (1) a collective of all the medicines having aggravation of any symptoms by warmth; 2] those having aggravation of any particular variety of symptoms (e.g., shooting) in any tissue (e.g., Bones) and 4] those having aggravatio of any variety of symptoms in each of these tissues. In this chapter doubtful symptoms are bracketed.

ABBREVIATION : Ciphering is used. The ciphers of the elements and simple haloid salts are the same as their chemical symbols; the – ate salts are ciphered by adding – I, to the cipher of the element or compound radicle from which they are formed. Thus Na. Sodium, Na-s. sulphide of sodium, Na–as sulphate of sodium, Na-si sulphite of sodium; s sulphur; s.x sulphuric acid; s.ix sulphurous acid; s.hx sulphydric acid.

GRADATION OF DRUGS :

First rank – Italic capitals *ARSENIC*

Second rank – plain capitals ARSENIC

Third rank – italics *Arsenic*

Fourth rank – Roman letters Arsenic

Doubtful drugs – Roman in brackets (Arsenic)

III. MINTONS UTERUS

Author: Henry Minton.

Year of Publication: **1883.**

Edition/Publication: 1995 Reprint Edition / B. Jain Publishers (Pvt) Ltd.

About the Author: Henry Minton is the famous author of "Diseases of Women and Children". He was also the Editor of "The Homeopathic Journal of Obstetrics and Diseases of Women and Children".

The "Uterine Therapeutics" is a useful monograph on the problems of menstruation and other related functions. It is a result of 16 years of patient study and clinical practice of the author. A large part of the symptomatology of the work was published in the "American Journal of Homeopathic Materia Medica, during the year 1874-75.

The aim of this repertory is to collect and arrange in a systematic and convenient form for ready reference all those symptoms of Materia Medica that have any direct or specific bearing upon the subject of uterine disorders.

Source Books of the Repertory: Minton has quoted Dr. Hovat in *Curare,* Dr.Hughes in *Glonoine* and even Dr.Hahnemann in *Dictamnus*. Other than their masterpieces he had also referred large number of books, records, journals, magazines and pamphlets for the making of this repertory.

Philosophical Background: The philosophy on which the construction and plan of this repertory is based are:

- Doctrine of Concomitants and Complete Symptoms : Like most of the Regional repertories, Minton's

therapeutics also emphasises on the importance of concomitants and complete symptoms.

- Doctrine of Causation and Time: Anyone who has gone through this book must have seen that each section of this repertory has a separate rubric of causation and time under it. This book gives importance to both these factors along with location, sensation modality and concomitant in dealing with a symptom.

- Evaluation of Remedies: Minton's Therapeutics also incorporates evaluation of remedies in its construction. The gradation is based on the frequency and intensity of the symptoms recorded.

- Clinical Rubrics: Being a Clinical Repertory this book has a record of a number of clinical conditions along with the group of medicines. This serves as a necessary aid in cases where there is advanced pathology or in paucity of symptom.

Plan and Construction: The arrangement of this repertory is based on "The Homeopathic Therapeutics of Diarrhoea" by James B.Bell. The credit for giving this book its present shape goes to the Editor, Dr. A.R.Thomas.

The Repertory starts with the quotes of Bacon and Horace. It is followed by the content under following headings:

- PREFACE - It was written on Sep1, 1883 in Brooklyn , New York . It is the story of how this book came into existence with a brief introduction of this book

- DEDICATION - It is dedicated to his friend E.T.Richardson

- LIST OF REMEDIES - This is a alphabetical record of all the medicines in this book with their abbreviations. The list includes 178 medicines from Aconite to Zingiber, though the actual number of medicines given is 177(Actea racemosa and Cimicifuga have been repeated)

PART I (MATERIA MEDICA) - This contains alphabetical arrangement of Medicines with their indications under the following headings -

o Menstruation.

o Before Menstruation.

o During Menstruation.

o After Menstruation.

o Amenorrhoea

o Metrorrhagia

o Lochia

o Leucorrhoea

o Concomitants (in general) this includes most of the important indications of the medicines, other than the uterine system. It also includes the mental picture of the medicine.

o Aggravation

o Amelioration

The last paragraph in most of the medicines deals with the adaptability of the medicine regarding- constitution, temperament, living conditions and even the disease conditions.

This part has been written with an aim to list for the practitioner all the necessary symptoms of the medicine. This section is a complete material medica in itself ready for use.

PART II (REPERTORY) – This section contains the Repertory Proper under the following headings –

- **Menstruation:** This section includes specifications of menses under:

  o Time and quantity of discharge.

  o Character of menstrual discharge.

  o Before menstruation.

  o During menstruation.

  o After menstruation

Basically this section has record of symptoms of menses. This section is very much similar in its content to the rubric "Menses" in other general repertories.

- **Amenorrhoea :** This section includes the rubrics:

  o **Cause and Concomitants:** It includes the causes most frequently associated with amenorrhoea along with the chief accompaniments.

- **Abortion - miscarriage:** This section includes the rubrics:

  o Cause

  o Character of the discharge.

  o Character of the pain.

  o Mental condition.

  o Metrorrhagia.

  o Character of the discharge.

  o Concomitants

This section gives rubrics describing the specifics of abortion. But the author has given Metrorrhagia under Abortion and not under Menstruation, though we know that Metrorrhagia is defined as profuse menses in quantity or in duration.

- **Lochia :** It includes:

  o Peculiarities of the discharge.

  o Concomitant symptoms.

This section deals with the change in character of Lochia which accompanies puerperal complaints.

- **Leucorrhoea:** It includes:
  o Character of the discharge.
  o Cause, Time, Aggravation and Amelioration of the discharge.
  o Concomitant symptoms.

This section deals with the peculiarities of leucorrhoea under the given rubrics.

- **General Concomitants:** This section covers the person as a whole from Mind to Generalities.
  o Mind and mood.
  o Sleep
  o Vertigo
  o Headache
  o Head
  o Eyes
  o Ears
  o Nose
  o Face
  o Mouth
  o Throat
  o Appetite
  o Eructations
  o Hiccough
  o Water brash
  o Nausea
  o Vomiting
  o Stomach
  o Abdomen
  o Anus
  o Rectun
  o Stool
  o Urination
  o Urine
  o Sexual organs
  o Sexual desire

o Mammae
o Nipples
o Chest
o Respiration
o Cough
o Heart
o Back
o Extremities
o Skin
o Persons - remedies especially suitable for
o Generalities

This section is a real marvel of this repertory. It includes separately and with details all parts of the body and their symptoms. It even includes parts of the female genitalia viz. Labia, Pudendum, Vulva, Vagina, Uterus, Ovaries both, Right, left etc. All the structural changes which could not be covered in the previous sections have been dealt with in this section.

Arrangement of Rubrics: Like most Regional Repertories of that time, the

- Rubrics in each chapter are in *Alphabetical* order
- Sub rubrics are given after an indentation followed by the medicines
- Sub sub rubrics are given with more indentation followed by a comma after each part

INDEX: At the end of the book Index has been given which has the sections and rubrics arranged alphabetically under it. This section facilitates the search of needed rubric.

Typographies Used: Two types of Typographies have been used in the whole book.

- Italics
- Ordinary Roman

Medicines are indicated in Part I (Materia medica) and Part II (Repertory) with same typographies.

Working out a case using Minton's Therapeutics:
The symptoms of the case to be worked out should be arranged in the following manner-

- Complaint
- Character of the discharge
- Cause
- Modalities
- Concomitant
- Generalities

In this way a complete picture of the case is formed, which can now be repertorised to choose the simillimum. The final choice can be confirmed using the Materia medica given in first part of the book.

Scope and Limitation of the Repertory :
Being a Regional Repertory, the scope of this repertory is for

- Cases lacking in Generals, but rich in Common symptoms.
- Cases with clinical diagnoses.
- Short cases with a few symptoms.

Howsoever, the rubrics given are result of clinical observations and so their use is limited to specific number of cases.

Merits of the Repertory :
- It is a very elaborate and detailed work covering most of the symptoms
- It contains rubrics related to females at one place, and so serves as a quick bed side reference.

- The section "Persons remedies especially for" is a masterpiece and covers most of the constitutions. It also serves as a confirmation stamp on the choice of remedy.
- Concomitant symptoms of each chapter are placed along with followed by general concomitant chapter in the end which contains symptoms of person as a whole.
- The General concomitant chapter contains the symptoms relating to the whole body and mind. It in itself forms a complete record of general symptoms.

Shortcomings of the Repertory :
- The number of medicines is limited.
- Being a clinical repertory, it is not complete and is mainly used for reference works.
- Same symptom is repeated under different rubrics or headings and again in concomitants.
- Mental condition is specifically given under "Abortion" only and not under "Amenorrhoea" or "Leucorrhoea". Though it is mentioned under General concomitants.
- Only: "Lochia" is given, no other complaint of pregnancy or lying-in-period is covered.
- Metrorrhagia is given under Abortion and not in Menses.
- Number of Clinical rubrics is also very limited.

In spite of the above shortcomings **Minton's Therapeutics** is a complete repertory in itself. The repertory can be used in most of the present female diseases with favorable results.

Author: DOUGLAS M. BORLAND M.B., Ch.B. (Glas.) FFHom. (1885 - 1960)

Year of Publication: 1939.

Edition/Publication: 2003 Reprint Edition / B. Jain Publishers Pvt Ltd.

About the Author: Dr Borland qualified MB, ChB at Glasgow University in 1909. After various hospital posts he went to Chicago to study under Dr Kent, going as an open-minded sceptic and returning as an astonished and convinced homoeopath. He then took an appointment at the London Homoeopathic Hospital, followed by active service during World War I with the Royal Army Medical Corps. After the war he established a consultant practice in London and returned to the staff of the London Homoeopathic Hospital, where he subsequently became senior consultant physician and chairman of the staff. He was respected for his presence as a doctor and his willingness to assist his colleagues. Borland was a pupil of Kent in 1908, he was one of those who brought Kentian philosophy to his motherland.

Borland wrote several popular books. These include:

Influenzas (1939)

Pneumonias (1939)

Children's Types (1939)

Some Emergencies of General Practice (1946)

Homeopathy for Mother and Infant (1950) Digestive Drugs

Homeopathy in Practice

Homeopathy in Theory and Practice Treatment of Certain Heart Conditions.

Borland died November 29, 1960.

About the Repertory: This book is part of shorthand notes of Postgraduate Lectures delivered by Dr. Borland at the London Homoeopathic Hospital (Reprinted from *Homoeopathy*). This lecture is a result of author's extensive experience on the subject. It contains not only the detailed therapeutics of Pneumonia but also a detailed discussion on the potency to be used and repetition of doses is given.

Aim of the Book: The aim of this book is to present in a concise manner the detailed knowledge of therapeutics and prescription of Pneumonias. This is a short booklet on the subject which helps the reader to deal with the case of Pneumonia and provide cure. Dr. Borland expected that when treating a pneumonia epidemic homeopathically there would be a 100% recovery rate.

Source of the Repertory: This book is part of shorthand notes of Postgraduate Lectures delivered by Dr. Borland at the London Homoeopathic Hospital (Reprinted from *Homoeopathy*).

Macroconstuction: The book is divided into two parts:

Part I: Understanding Pneumonia with remedies and their Indications.

Part II: Repertory

Contents with page number

Part I : The first part of the book aims at knowing Pneumonia from homoeopathic view. The salient features which Dr. Borland has tried to deal with in the first part are:

- Prescription should be based on Totality of symptoms covering the disease picture as well as the patient picture

- To recognize difference between pathognomic and non pathognomic symptoms. Prescription should always be based on non pathognomic symptoms and not on pathognomic symptoms which Borland called as diagnostic symptoms.

- For a perfect cure, physician should choose: Right medicine; Right strength of drug i.e. potency and Right repetition of drug.

- Role of potencies

  *In Acute disease if you restrict your prescription to **low potencies** you avoided the complications of the disease, you made your patients more comfortable and you reduced your mortality rate. But by this method you do not reduce the duration of disease.*

  *By the administration of **higher potencies**, - something above 30 you will find that you abort the disease. It does not run its normal course; the duration of the illness is very much shortened and you have an anticipated crisis.*

- For Repetition of doses

  *When you are using **low potencies**, you have to keep up your drug administration right throughout the course of the disease. When you are using the **higher potencies**, it is advisable to continue the administration of the selected drug until the temperature has reached normal and has remained normal for at least 6 hours.*

In average case where you are using a low potency it is quite sufficient to give the drug about once in four hours. As far as the high potencies are concerned, I think it is wiser to give the drug every 2 hours, the reason being that you want a number of stimuli in a comparatively short period of time in order to obtain the crisis within 12-24 hours.

Dr. Borland also advocates that *'Many people advocate that at the start it is wiser to use low potencies until you acquire confidence in your selection and then as you gain greater knowledge heighten the potency and shorten the interval, so that eventually you are treating all your crisis with medium or high potency.*

Personally, I think it is better to go out for the best right from the start'

- Understanding the **Stages of Disease and group of the Homeopathic drugs** which would cover each stage.

Associating drugs according to symptoms presented in clinical practice.

Group I Incipient Stage

(Aconite, Belladona, Ferrrum-phos, Ipecac)

In each drug, description of picture of patient during onset, attack is given. Like peculiarities of Aconite patient in Incipient stage, Choice of potency, action of potency and the changes it produces is explained.

Group II Frankly developed Pneumonia

After the first 24 hours consider Bryonia, Phosphorus, Veratrum-viride and Chelidonium. Bryonia is consider in milder weather while Phosphorus in colder weather.

In the first part description of each drug is given in detail and in the second part the Directions for choosing Dosage is given.

Developed Pneumonia: Use of high potencies CM, 10M.

Frankly developed Pneumonia: At least 6 doses of medicine. One finds that the average length of action of action of each dose is around 2 hours; 6 doses of whatever potency probably a 10M and repeat every 2 hours.

Group III - Complicated Pneumonia
Mixed patient or unhealthy patient

- Creeping type of Pneumonia or Frank Broncho-pneumonia

A) *Mixed patient or Alcoholic patient: Baptisia, Mercurius, Rhus-tox, Pyrogen, Hepar-sulph, Lachesis (Lachesis is the most commonly used drug at this stage):* Picture of patient is given.

B) *Creeping type of Pneumonia, or Definite Bronchopneumonia in Adult: Pulsatilla, Natrum-sulph, Senega and Lobelia.* Picture of patient is given.

The best potency at this stage was a 1M, which seemed to be high but not dangerous. In Frankly alcoholic patient with pneumococcal infection give high potency.

Group IV Late Pneumonia: *One that is not resolving well, not clearing up satisfactorily. Antim-tart, Carbo-veg, Kali-carb, Ars-alb, Lycopodium, Sulph.*

Picture of the patient along with choice of potency is given. For example:

Carbo-veg: CM's every 10 or 15 minute.

Lycopodium: 10M's 2 hourly.

Sulphur CM's 2 hourly.

Part II: Therapeutic Symptom Index

This part contains a symptom index of the first part of the book.

Microconstuction

1. The second part is divided into 21 sections or chapters consisting of:

General.

Mentals

Head and Vertigo

Face and Lips

Mouth

Tongue

Eyes

Nose

Throat

Stomach

Abdomen

Rectum

Chest

Cough

Sputum

Heart

Pulse

Temperature

Extremities

Skin

Sleep

Chapters are arranged following Hahnemann's schema. The first chapter is General (containing stages, onset, temperature reactions, weather)

2. The Rubrics are written in Roman case arranged alphabetically.

3. Subrubrics- are written in Italic case starting with an indent and also arranged alphabetically.

4. Medicines are listed in each rubric, subrubric alphabetically followed by the page number where it is mentioned.

5. Cross reference are mentioned in (brackets, after See.)

Total number of Medicines: 24.

How to use the Repertory: Dr. Borland explained the implementation of his therapeutic index in the first part:

"Suppose you take a case of pneumonia; it does not interest you that the patient has a temperature, a rapid pulse, rapid respiration, rusty sputum, because all the drugs you consider for the treatment of a pneumonia have these symptoms and you do not need to bother about them at all.

"But it does matter to you whether the individual patient has a generally evenly coated tongue, whether he has a dry mouth or a moist one, whether he is thirsty or thirstless, whether he is more comfortable lying on the affected side or on the opposite one, whether he is drugged and toxic or delirious and excited, whether he is more at peace with somebody by his bed or prefers to be left alone.

"All that sort of thing you very definitely want to know; it is on that sort of thing you prescribe; but you only take it into account after you have decided that the drugs you are considering have the constant features on which you have made your diagnosis.

"It is not a question of neglecting your clinical side; it is a question of knowing which drugs have the clinical picture, and adding to that the points on which you are going to prescribe."

ADVANTAGES:

1. In some symptoms i.e. those related to Pneumonia, care has been taken to form a complete symptom for example
   Chapter: Chest
     Rubric: Pain
       Area affected:
       Aggravated by:
       Ameliorated by:
   Chapter: Cough
     Rubric: Aggravated by:
       Ameliorated by:

2. Rubric describing the physical type of patient is also given, under Generals
   (Type physical) which helps in forming the totality.

3. Pathological rubrics like consolidation, Pain: pleuritic have been included.

4. A special rubric for deciding the thermal reaction of patiens is given. Rubric: Temperature reaction to: Sensitive to cold (for Chilly); Sensitive to heat (for Hot); Sensitive to heat and cold (for Ambithermal).

5. Special rubrics related to mind have been included like: Desires hand being held, Dislike of particular person, Interference resents, Unpleasant occurences relates.

6. Handy and concise.

7. Contains rubrics related to Pneumonia with concomitants at one place.

8. Quick prescription in case of pneumonia at any stage.

DISADVANTAGES:

1. Limited number of rubrics.
2. NO GRADATION OF REMEDIES
3. Number of remedies is very less.

Comments: 'Borland's Pneumonia' is more of a treatise on the subject than a repertory. No doubt it has long been known for its repertorial part, but it is more of an Index than a repertory. In the first chapter of General we have rubrics for potency, repetition of doses which is unusual considering it as repertory on Pneumonia. Also there is no gradation of remedies, so the book serves for quick prescription instead of proper repertorisation.

Dr. Borland is famous for his booklets wherein he extensively described the indications of medicines in the condition, ending the booklet with a short alphabetic index. Even his book on 'Influenzas' deals with the medicines indicated followed by an index. Though in this book the description of index is elaborate but it lacks precision if compared to other regional repertories.

So 'Borland's Pneumonia' can be thought of as a treatise on Pneumonia identifying stages of disease, its symptoms, related medicines, potency to be prescribed and repetition needed.

Dr. William. A. Allen prepared his Repertory to the symptoms of intermittent fever mainly for two reasons:

1] He had many cases under his professional care.

2] Many physicians and laymen asserted that Homoeopathic treatment is totally unable to suppress the paroxysm, to remove the pathological conditions and symptoms incident to them - to cure.

This repertory was published in 1882.

Dr. Allen says that absolutely certainly these things can be cured without any exception and that to succeed, it is only necessary to administer a remedy of proper potency selected in accordance with the law of similia, having in its choice a regard for the totality of symptoms.

Dr. T. F. Allen writes that Allens Repertory is exceedingly valuable. It should be printed in pocket form, I should use it constantly. He further says that Dr.Allen has a large experience in the treatment of intermittent. And his own observations are entitled to great respect.

While compiling this repertory Dr. Allen has referred the following books — The Homoeopathic therapeutics of intermittent fever, by Dr. H.C.Allen, Lippes Repertory, Boenninghausen's Therapeutics, Gross on comparative Materia Medica. To these he had added such symptoms as have come to his notice in the treatment of these cases.

Construction

Symptoms are arranged under 4 main headings :

1] **Chill**

2] **Heat**

3] **Sweat**

4] **Symptoms during apyrexia**

With a small heading of remedies special indications for and season and weather (which are given in the chill).

CHILL

Symptoms during chill stage are given in relation to following headings:

A] Chill caused by

B] Chill preceded by

C] Time of chill

D] Commencement of chill

E] Location of chill

F] Character of chill

G] Symptoms during chill

H] Chill ameliorated

I] Chill aggravated

J] Chill followed by

HEAT

A] Heat proceeded by

B] Heat — character, time, and location of heat

C] Heat symptoms during

D] Heat ameliorated

E] Heat aggravated

F] Heat followed by

SWEAT:

A] Sweat preceded by

B] Sweat, character and time of

C] Location of sweat

D] Symptoms during sweat

E] Sweat ameliorated

F] Sweat aggravated

G] Sweat followed by

SYMPTOMS DURING APYREXIA

All the symptoms that are observed during apyrexial period are given under this heading in alphabetical order.

Number of remedies 133

Grades —3 BOLD

2 - Italics

1 - Roman

Regarding the potency to be used he says that he has used from Q to hundred-thousandths potency but he recommends that remedies may be used two hundred upwards.

The best time to begin to administer the remedy is after the height of the paroxysm has been passed. This is particularly true of Nat. M.

Regarding the repetition he says — there is no doubt about efficacy of single dose, which he has used in number of cases but I some cases he has continued the medicine for several days after the paroxysm has ceased.

VI. THERAPEUTICS OF INTERMITTENT FEVER BY H. C. ALLEN

Name of book: Therapeutics of intermittent fever.

Author : H.C. Allen, MD. Author of Keynotes and characteristic of materia medica, materia medica of nosodes, and therapeutics of fever.

Classification: Coming under the category – clinical repertory on the clinical condition intermittent fever.

Publishers : B. Jain Publishers Pvt .Ltd, New Delhi (India).

Edition & year: First edition 1879 of publication Second edition 1884 Reprint edition 1998.

Total number on pages: 342 pages (including Materia medica part) 82 pages repertory alone.

Grading : Bold, italics, and ordinary letters

Mode of construction of book:

The book can be divided into five parts.

Preface

There are two prefaces given in this book one for the first edition and the other for the second edition.

INTRODUCTION

Begins with a coating from Hahnemann's "medicine of experience". " After he has found all the existing and appreciable symptoms of the disease, the physician has found the disease itself. He has a complete idea of it and knows all he need know to cure it".

Introduction consists of few important essays.

These essays include

"The cause", "Malarial theory", "Psoric diathesis", "Examination of the patient", "Genus epidemicus" etc.

Materia Medica part — given as two sections.

First section begins with Aconite and ends with Veratrum album. This part consists of 116 medicines.

Second part given under the heading "minor remedies". This part consists of 31 medicines. Begins with Aethusa and ends with Valariana.

Total number of medicines in materia medica part is 147.

Repertory

Begins with – Chill– Type and ends with the chapter Apyrexia

Abbreviation and remedies

Materia Medica:

General representation of a medicine is as follows-

Name of medicine

General characteristics of medicine (both mental and physical)

Relation – Complimentary, acute, chronic, inimical etc

Aggravation

Modality

Amelioration

Followed by nature of fever described under the heading

1. Type (of fever)—Quotidian, tertian, yellow fever, typhoid etc.
2. Time –12 – 2 am, 2 – 4 am etc.
3. Prodrome
4. Chill
5. Heat
6. Sweat
7. Tongue
8. Pulse
9. Apyrexia

Comparison – Under certain drug like Ars alb, Capsicum etc. a comparative study of most similar drug is given. E.g.:- in drug Capsicum; Eup. purp. compared with capsicum. in drug Ars alb; Cinchona compared with Ars alb. Analysis – under analysis he mentioned most important characteristic symptoms of the drug in fever.

[Causation / important features of chill, heat and sweat etc].

Clinical - a separate clinical section is given at the end of each drug where examples of cases treated either by him or by others with that drug are mentioned.

Plan of construction of repertory
The mode of construction and the arrangement is the same as that in the " Therapeutics of fever" by the same author. One new feature is added to this work in the sub rubric level. Instead of repeating each word of main rubrics, the sub rubric begins with small lines (...), which indicate the words in the preceding line. It contains 147 medicines and has 31 chapter starts with " chill-type" and ends with the chapter apyrexia symptoms during.

The repertory part can be divided in to 5 sections
1. Chill
2. Heat
3. Sweat
4. Appetite, taste, tongue etc. Symptoms of
5. Apyrexia.

A) *Chill consists of 10 chapters. They are as follows*
1. Type
2. Time
3. Cause (attack brought on by)
4. Prodrome (conditions occurring during)
5. Commencement of chill (chill beginning in)
6. Chill location of (chill part affected or location of)
7. Chill aggravated
8. Chill ameliorated
9. Symptoms during the chill
10. Chill followed by

B) *Heat consists of 7 chapters.*
1. Heat aggravated by
2. Heat ameliorated by
3. Heat absent
4. Heat in general
5. Heat symptoms during
6. Heat followed by
7. Heat character of

C) *Sweat –11 chapters.*
1. Sweat aggravated
2. Sweat ameliorated
3. Sweat followed by

4. Sweat absent
5. Sweat in general
6. Sweat predominate
7. Sweat produced by
8. Sweat character of
9. Sweat time of
10. Sweat location of
11. Sweat symptoms during

D) *Appetite, taste, tongue etc. Symptoms of*

E) *Apyrexia symptoms during*

Merits:

No repetition of same rubrics as in the case of therapeutics of fever.

It contains many additional rubrics when compared to other repertories.

E.g.: – Chill location of
- Abdomen
- Arms
- Arm left
- Back, in, or on the etc

Cause
- Mechanical injuries from
- Organic lesion

Whole febrile condition is divided in to four stages i.e. chill, heat, sweat and apyrexia. Each of this stage further subdivided into type, time, location of, cause etc. There by the selection of the rubrics become more accurate and easier.

Demerits:

- Misplaced rubrics are many.
- No definite pattern or order for the arrangement different chapters.
- Number of medicines is less when compared to Murphy or other modern repertory.
- Even though grading is given as bold, Italics and ordinary letters, there is no information about it s mark.
- Rubrics are given in alphabetical order but in some places order is not followed.
- Eg: under the chapter "Chill- type" the rubric- Fever, without chill, returning at is given in wrong alphabetical order.
- Under the section chill, there were two chapters with the same heading with entirely different rubrics. i.e. "symptoms during the chill" and "chill, symptoms during"
- No index for this work
- No introduction for repertory part.
- Name of the chapter is given only at the beginning of each chapter, not given in subsequent page top. It makes some difficulties in search of rubrics

Repertories became voluminous and more complex with the introduction of new philosophies and different types of constructions. The practitioners found it difficult to put them into day-to-day practice. Few of them found that if the rubrics in the books were written on separate pieces of paper, one could quickly glance through them and find simillimum. They started to prepare their own chits, diaries and different paper cuttings. These efforts finally gave birth to Card Repertories.

- Rubrics were written on separate pieces of paper – to quickly glance through them – to save time and energy.

- People prepared their own chits, diaries and paper cuttings – birth of card repertories.

- Card repertories have several cards with rubrics written on top with a group of medicines below.

Card repertory is a system of visual sorting which helps the physician by eliminating the necessity of writing out the rubrics and remedies against them.

MERITS

- One has to select the cards according to rubrics arranged in repertorial totality and look for common remedies

- It saves time as compared to manual writing down. It cuts down time needed in calculation of marks and analysis

- It does not require paper work

- Purpose – elimination of remedies in reportorial analysis

DEMERITS

- It is difficult to list all remedies and all medicines.

- Most of the card repertories do not represent the rubrics well, especially sub-rubrics. It is difficult to use finer expressions at general and particular levels in repertorisation.

- Computers have made it obsolete.

METHOD OF WORKING OUT A CASE

In this, symptoms are converted into rubrics. The rubrics are seen in the index book, to look for the particular card number. The rubric were chosen from the index and the indicated slips were taken out and made to lie side by side so that name of each remedy ran in a straight line from left to right, on adding up the exponent of several remedies, one with the highest number is the possible remedy for the case.

PRINCIPLES OF CONSTRUCTION

- Important generals are used as rubrics

- Numerical evaluation plays a little role in this method

- Cards are employed to determine the likely group of remedies that closely correspond to the general picture of the case

- It usually suits to a chronic case, which presents with a changed but vivid symptoms

SELECTION OF RUBRICS

- Conversion of the symptoms in to rubrics should be accurate
- Characteristic concomitant must be always included
- Top priority should be given to the cause
- Generalization of a particular symptom on inadequate grounds should be avoided

REQUISITES OF A GOOD CARD REPERTORY

- Most card reps were limited in scope due to improper construction
- Too small and give only a broad general selection limited to few polychrests
- Most important use is ELIMINATIVE FUNCTION

1. Results should be as close as possible to factual texts on repertory.
2. Cards should be of standard texture and thinness.
3. Should be strong as well as thin enough and should not shut off light completely
4. Punching should follow standard methods
5. Card system should be elastic, so that new rubrics can be introduced or new remedies added
6. Punching should indicate degree of drugs.

EVOLUTION

1888	W J Guernsey	Guernsey's	2500 cards1.25 inch X
1892	Improved by H C Allen	Boenninghausen's Slips	12.5 inch.
1912	Margaret Tyler	Punched Card Repertory Based on Kent	1000 cards
1913	Welch & Houston	Loose Punched Card Repertory Based on Kent's Generals	134 cards
1922	Field	Field's Card Repertory Based on Kent and Boger	6800 cards360 drugs
1928	Boger	Boger's Card Index Repertory Foreword by L D Dhawale	
1948	Marcos Jaminez	Based on Boenninghausene	600 larg cards
1910	Enrique Jaminez		Introduced evaluation of drugs
	Braussalian	Card RepertoryBased on Kent	1861 cards640 drugs
1950	J G Weiss	Card Repertory	
	Farley	Spindle Card Repertory	
	Young & Pulford	Not published	
	L D Dhawale	Modified Boger's cards Not published	

1950	P Sankaran	Card RepertoryBased on Boger's Card Repertory	420 cards292 drugs
1959	Jugal Kishore	Kishore Card Repertory	10000 cards
1984	Shashi Mohan Sharma	Based on Kent's Final Repertorium Generale	3000 cards

FEW IMPORTANT CARD REPERTORIES:

GUERNSEY'S BOENNINGHAUSEN'S SLIPS

- Prepared by William Jefferson Guernsey, nephew of H. N. Guernsey
- Prepared in 1888, released in 1892.
- Chapman called it "Perfection of method for managing MM."
- Long cards or slips – 1.25 inch X 12.5 inch
- 2500 cards; 126 remedies
- On each card was printed in alphabetical order, names of remedies used in Boenninghausen's work
- On top was code number of rubric
- A separate index with coded rubrics
- On each card, remedies had number 1 to 4 printed against them, depending upon degree of evaluation of that drug according to TPB.
- Rubrics were chosen from index and the slips made to lie side by side, so that name of each remedy ran in a straight line from left to right.

H C Allen improved the original slips by adding more remedies and were known as Allen's Boenninghausen's Slips.

MARGARET TYLER'S PUNCHED CARD REPERTORY

- Made in 1912, but discouraged by Kent
- Used large cards and hand punched them
- Based on Kent
- Incomplete work
- 1000 cards

FIELD'S CARDS

- Made in 1922
- Included Kent's rubrics as well few from others.
- Included Boger's and Skinner's corrections and annotations
- 6800 cards + 360 remedies with a provision for 40 more
- Only first and second grade remedies were punched
- Was the first to code names of remedies into numbers
- Cards were thick and blocked the remedy easily

BOGER'S CARD INDEX REPERTORY

- Published in 1928
- Consists of 339 cards + 224 drugs?
- One rubric per card – CIRCULAR PUNCHES

- Fewer rubrics are used; more stress on pathological generals than disease diagnosis – bluish, convulsive, cough, albuminous discharges, dryness, rawness
- Rubrics for prominent mental conditions are also included – anger, fearsome, excitement
- Clinical symptoms are first divided into 'General' or constitutional characteristics. The perforated cards covering these rubrics placed in apposition and held up to light.
- Hayes suggested a method of working with the Card Index.

ADVANTAGES

- When closely competing remedies have missing symptoms, this helps to decide easily
- It is of special value in working out cases having a paucity of symptoms
- Boger united in one rubric various influences or conditions and this has made it quick and safe

MARCOZ JIMENEZ COLOURED CARD REPERTORY

In 1948, **Dr. Marcoz Jimenez** introduced practical Homeopathic Repertory in colored and perforated cards. This Repertory was published at Maxica, 126 pages. The Repertory contains 552 cards and 480 remedies. Each card is divided into 480 little squares. Each square was numbered and represented a remedy. Whichever drug was in agiven rubric that particular square representing drug was punched.

Gradation: 3 marks – square coloured red, 2 marks – square coloured blue, 1 mark – square uncoloured. Based on rubrics from Kent's repertory.

Different sections have different colors; the mind section is on yellow cards, while the mouth, ear, nose, and throat are on blue cards. Once the required cards are given in a given case were selected, the cards were superimposed and held against light. Perforations common to all cards were noted and the drugs representing the perforated squares were considered fo r further differentiation to reach similimum.

This comes in a cedar box along with cards is a pocket manual written in Spanish and English, which explains method of evaluation of symptoms, process and techniques of repertory.

P. SANKARAN'S POCKET CARD REPERTORY

- 420 cards – last card is numbered 392, as there are a number of cards marked 'A' in between, eg 45A, 89A
- Each card carries abbreviated names of 292 remedies
- In each card, punches are made below those drugs that cover the symptom – RECTANGULAR PUNCHES.
- Characteristics selected – Index to Card Rep referred – cards are picked and put together in apposition – group of remedies selected – reference to MM and bigger reps.
- Has more remedies and more comprehensive rubrics; remedies are better presented and provides numerous cross references.

Card size-7.4by 2.2inches 27 verticle by 12 horizontal columns ,420 cards.punchin in small, rectangular holes, booklet-name of rubrics acc to numberz n name of medicines, used in acute n chronic, kent's plus boenninghausen's concept.

SHASHI MOHAN'S CARDS

In 1984 **Dr.S.M.Sharma** prepared and published his card Repertory based on Kent's Work with 3000 cards and 400 remedies. Dr. Shashi Mohan Sharma's card Repertory is based on Kent's Repertory published by B. Jain Publication in 1984. Like Jugal Kishores Card Repertory, in this Repertory also majority of the General Rubrics are considered from Kent's Repertory.

The card of S.M. Sharma's Card Repertory is approx. 3½ x 7½. Author has selected 400 remedies for Inclusion in this card Repertory. The numbers of Rubrics (Cards) are 3,000 arranged alphabetically. Each card is designed same as Jugal Kishores card except those 4 vertical columns which are reserved for rubric number.

Remedies are arranged in 40 vertical columns i.e. 40 x 10 = 400. First number starts from 10 and the vertical columns are numbered from 0 to 9. At the bottom the serial number of horizontal rooms are recorded from 1 to 40. Remedies are punched in the rooms, which are indicated for recorded rubric on the top.

PATWARDHAN'S CARD REPERTORY

Dr. Patwardhan's card Repertory published his card Repertory. Dr. A. B. Patwardhan from PUNE, Maharashtra prepared card Repertory called "Homoeo. Card Deck" is the card Repertory consists of two parts –

1) Cards. 2) Booklet.

There are 1245 cards in his card Repertory. For rubrics 299 remedies have been made use of Punches representing remedies for the particular rubric are present. A serial number of the card is printed on the right hand corner. On the top of each card is printed the rubrics or symptoms the card represents. There are thus 1245 rubrics represented separately on 1245 cards.

The punches beyond 76 up to 79 denote the serial number of the card and may not be confused for the indications of any remedy. With the 'Card-deck', standard card bearing all 299 remedies at their proper place are supplied which can be superimposed and the names of the Remedies at their respectable places can be easily read out. One side of the card is printed while the other side is blank.

THE KISHORE CARDS – A HOMOEOPATHIC CARD REPERTORY

By Dr. Jugal Kishore and Dr. Arvind Kishore.

First Edition: 1959

Second Revised and Enlarged Edition: 1967

Third and Enlarged Edition: 1985

CONTENTS

Part I: **Introduction**

Part II: **Rubrics and their code numbers**

It took about seven years to complete the first edition of the Card Repertory. About 579 medicines and 3497 rubrics were included in the repertory. The rubrics are arranged in the alphabetical order and they are numbered from 50.

There are certain remedies, which do not appear under any of the rubrics; are included and assigned code number, so as to enable practitioner to add such remedies in suitable rubrics; when his experience and study dictate their inclusion. Most of the rubrics from Kent's and Boenninghausen's Repertories were included in this repertory. The repertory is so constructed that a Practitioner can use it either according to the Boenninghausen method or Kent method. Information from about 91 books was included in this card repertory.

These cards are primarily meant for quick elimination of remedies without the risk of excluding simillimum. The elimination is a mechanical process. The rubric number is stamped on the top of each card. For quick reference a table of contents of some important rubrics are given at the beginning of index. Cross-references are also given. Meanings of some rubrics are also given. For example; code number 1570 – Fever: Zymotic. The meaning of Zymotic has been given within brackets – Fever due to specific virus.

For evaluating remedies he has used two types of holes; round/ square holes and oval/ figure of eight holes. The latter indicate the high grade and the former indicate the lower grade remedies.

WORKING METHOD:

After case taking, the rubrics are arranged in the descending order of their importance. "Red line" rubrics are considered at the upper most. The respective code numbers are written against each other rubrics. Then pick out the cards for the corresponding numbers, put them in the order of the list; one behind the other, leaving aside (for the time being) the cards of less importance or those rubrics with very few remedies. After arrangement; look for the synchronizing of the holes. Not more than three holes could be seen through the upper most (first) card. He notes down the holes of the cards. Decode those remedy numbers; by using the code numbers and list of remedies. We can also note down the second group of remedies which are not all through but are

most tarns -illuminant. In certain cases, there may not be any hole going through the all the cards. In such cases, the most illuminant holes should be noted down and decoded. There is an isolated punched hole at the top of left corner of the card. It is only meant for checking and does not have any significance.

In the second edition, the number of rubrics increased to 9063 and the number of medicine increased to 590.

In the third edition, 129 new rubrics and 102 new remedies were added. So that the total number of rubrics in the third edition is 9192 and the total number of remedies is 692. Jugal Kishore's son Arvind Kishore has given his contributions in this edition.

Description of the 'Rubric card' (Kishore Cards)

A card has 80 vertical columns; numbering from 1 to 80 from left to right. They are numbered at the bottom and top in small type. Each vertical column from above downwards contains number from 0 to 9. The first four vertical columns are kept apart (without being divided by vertical lines). They are meant for punching the number of rubric. The rest of the vertical columns are meant for the coded remedies, which have these particular symptoms. The remedies are indicated by the punched holes. The punched number (any number from 0 to 9) is placed against the small digit number placed at the bottom or top of the column; containing that particular hole and that gives us the number of the remedy. The remedy can be made out from the list of ' Remedies and their code numbers'. The code number of remedies starts from 50. The total number of remedies that can be punched on this card is 800; but since we are utilizing first four columns for the number of rubric, the available space on the card is only for 750 remedies. On the top of the card is printed the name of the rubric along with its code number.

MERITS

1. Third edition contains 692 medicines and 9192 rubrics

2. Almost all rubrics in the Kent's repertory are incorporated in the Card repertory

3. This repertory can be used in two methods, Kent's and Boenninghausen.

4. Many of the rubrics in the Boenninghausen's repertory are made available, up to date and complete.

5. Elimination is a mechanical process. We can save the time taken for writing down all the rubrics, medicines and adding their marks. Hence useful for very busy Practitioners

6. The rubrics and the cards are arranged in alphabetical order; so easy to find the required rubric. Table of contents of rubrics with their code numbers is given in the index.

7. Contents of the medicines with their code numbers are given in the index

8. Cross-references are helpful in finding the related and similar rubrics

9. Evaluation of medicines can be done with changing the shape of the holes

10. New remedies are added from the reliable source like British Homoeopathic Journal

11. It requires no paper work

12. It is useful in rural areas were Electricity and computers are not available.

DEMERITS

1. Quite voluminous (Repertory include three boxes of cards)

2. Not all rubrics needed in day to day practice will not be available in the card repertory

3. A thorough knowledge of rubrics are necessary before starting the process of repertorisation

4. Evaluation of remedies require an additional amount

5. There are certain medicines in the list , which are not found under any of the rubrics

6. With the invention of computer software repertories, card repertories become out dated.

0 MUSCLES, PAIN, STITCHING

DR SHASHI MOHAN SHARMA'S
HOMOEOPATHIC
CARD REPERTORY

IDM 1722 PRINTED IN INDIA

A. SYNTHESIS REPERTORY

Full name of the repertory: Repertorium Homoeopathicum Syntheticum.

Author: Dr. Frederik Schroyens. He was born in January 12, 1953 in Mechelen, Belgium. Schroyens is a 1977 medical graduate of the State University of Gent (Belgium) and a 1978 graduate of the one-year Homeopathic Training Course at the Faculty for Homeopathy in London (MFHom). Dr. Schroyens was one of the first RADAR users in 1986 and became enthusiastic about the increasing possibilities computer science offers to Homeopathy. Because of his dedication to the program, he became the Homeopathic Co-ordinator of the RADAR Project.

ORIGIN OF WORD 'SYNTHESIS'

From Greek word syntithenai – to put together; from syn + tithenai to put, place.

First Known Use: **1589.**

MEANING OF 'SYNTHESIS'

- The process of putting together separate parts to form a complete whole.

- Making a whole out of parts.

- The combination of separate elements in a whole.

SYNTHESIS is nothing but the on going process of collection and compilation of symptoms converted into rubrics with corresponding medicines and their gradations from various sources.

WHY 'SYNTHESIS'

Changes are taking place in all walks of life, all over the world. A system which is immune to change cannot stand for a long period of time. Each system should uphold the changes happening in the environment and adjust itself to the changing condition, so that, it can make the system vital. Absence of such changing will hamper our system. But it is clear to all of us that changing should be constructive one and without compromising on our basic principles.

HISTORY BEHIND

Repertories are developed to help the homoeopathic doctors in comparative study of materia media and in indicating some group of similar medicines to a given case.

Since, Hahnemann, who first felt the necessity of repertory, till date we have many repertories available in the market. In this regard, we must not forget Clemens von Boenninghausen, who first created the usable repertory in 1832.

Different authors expanded on previous versions of this repertory, e.g. T. F. Allen (1880; *Symptom Register*), Jahr (1835; *Symptom Repertory*), Lippe (1854; *A Repertory of Comparative Materia Medica*). Some created completely new structures as did Gentry (1890; *The Repertory of Concordance*) and Knerr (1896; *The Repertory to Hering's Guiding Symptoms*).

The glory of development of repertory came to its pick by the publication of Kent's repertory fascicle by fascicle from 1897 to 1899. For a few decades, no other repertories succeeded in taking up the challenge of progress after the publication of successive editions of Kent's repertory. But later on after the 6th edition of Kent's repertory in 1957 several Indian editions have been printed, which contain an unacceptable amount of mistakes. In this regard we have the comment of Dr. George Vithoulkas in foreword to the Synthesis Version 5. He says- "Kent's repertory, even if it is the best so far, contains a lot of errors; its structure and its logic are not always maintained, etc. I felt there was no good reason to reprint all the same errors once more, even with lot of additions, because this was done already too often by other so called new repertories."

It was the era of development and publication of new repertories by different authors mainly based upon the Kent's philosophy. These new repertories are still coming with some modifications and additions. Repertories like Synthetic (1973), Synthesis (1987), Murphy (1993; Indian edition 1994), Complete (1996) etc. are the fruits of this new era.

In 1973, Barthel and Klunler started the publication of a 1st version of their 'Synthetic Repertory', adding information from 14, later from 16 authors to the five (5) main chapters of the repertory (Mind, Generals, Sleep & Dreams, Male and Female Sexuality). They did not expand their work to more authors or chapters; their repertory was considered a new reference by many.

So it was this background that we needed a new, more complete, informative repertory to overcome the pitfalls of previous repertories.

Dr. Frederik Schroyens ultimately did this job in collaboration with the leading homoeopaths throughout the world leading to the development of synthesis repertory. Synthesis is a repertory linked to RADAR (Rapid Aid to Drug Aimed Research) project. It is based on 6th American edition of Kent's repertory and contains all its rubrics and remedies. Since 1987 Synthesis has been used as database for RADAR. It has been commented upon and there by improved over and over again. Indeed not only additions of an increasing number of authors but also correction of existing data have been integrated.

EVOLUTION OF SYNTHESIS REPERTORY

Synthesis is the product of a continuous teamwork with superb technology. It is the printed version of RADAR computer programme. This repertory has set a new standard by adding many information and continuous verification by its users. It is the latest among all repertories. Synthesis repertory is based on 6th American edition of Kent's repertory, and contains all its rubrics and remedies maintaining its philosophical background also. The synthesis repertory linked to the RADAR project. RADAR was first developed as research project at the University of Namur (Belgium) under the supervision of Jean Fichefet. He was the professor of mathematics in the department of computer science at the same university. He became interested in homoeopathy after the miraculous cure of his son by homoeopathic medicine. Dr. Frederik Schroyens became the homoeopathic co-ordinator for the

RADAR project. He had outlined a request for collaboration in the year 1986. Dr. Frederik Schroyens and his team sent charter to all leading homoeopaths who were concerned with evolution of homoeopathy through the software version. Since 1987 Synthesis is used as a database software programme, i.e. RADAR in daily practice of leading homoeopaths. This book is primarily based on 6th edition of Kent's repertory and has been commented upon and improved from time to time by various leading practitioners worldwide.

DIFFERENT VERSIONS AND THEIR PUBLICATIONS

- Version 1- In 1987; Synthesis was used as database for RADAR project.
- Version 2- In April, 1988. (10.5 MB was released).
- Version 3- In September, 1990. (11.5 MB was released). This version contains 136000 additions from 130 authors compared to Kent's original repertory.
- Version 4- In December, 1992. It contains 178000 additions from 200 authors.
- Synthesis 5x- German edition was published in August, 1993. English edition was published in February, 1994. Indian edition in March, 1996. Dutch edition in April, 1994, with only 'Mind' chapter. *This version was first time printed as book form*.
- Synthesis 6- German edition in August, 1995.
- Synthesis 7.1- English edition in July, 1997. It contains 235000 additions from 330 different sources.
- Synthesis 8.0- In February, 2002. It has 3031 author references and 4200 medicine references.

- Synthesis 9.0- In November, 2003.
- Synthesis 9.1- In June, 2004.

Synthesis treasure edition: The synthesis treasure edition was released as software in English and German on February, 2007. The French version was released in March, 2006. This edition is called treasure edition as the Synthesis repertory now includes Kent's "Lost Treasure" — 11,398 additions and corrections that were noted by Kent in his personal copies of his Repertory, plus 333 handwritten additions taken from his copy of Hering's Guiding Symptoms.

ENHANCEMENT OF THE QUALITY OF SYNTHESIS REPERTORY

At each edition or version of Synthesis the quality has improved as it is quite evident from the data that there was a 24% increase in new information from Synthesis 2 to Synthesis 3, and there was a 30% increase in new information from Synthesis 3 to Synthesis 4. In Synthesis 4 software version (December 1992) contains 178,000 additions to Kent's repertory from about 2,000 reliable sources. Publication of Synthesis 5 was a milestone as it was the first printed version. Synthesis shows a drastic increase in quality of repertory considering its structure, language and information. In further versions also synthesis went on improving its exclusive quality on the basis of maintaining following criteria:

- By doing corrections in the basic repertories (Kent's repertory) in a systematic manner.
- Different persisting symptoms are edited in more comprehensive format.
- Different words are modified by adding many new rubrics and new remedies after repeated verifications.
- Adding synonyms and cross references.

PHILOSOPHY

It is based on the sixth American edition of Kent's Repertory and contains all its rubrics and remedies. Therefore this repertory maintains the philosophy of Kent i.e. concept of individualization through evaluation of symptoms, evaluation of symptoms following deductive logic, gradation of medicine & it's basis, cross references etc. This repertory is the best example of the expanded version of Kent's Repertory from 1916 till date. It retains the hierarchical structure; therefore there is no need to learn a new format.

PLAN OF CONSTRUCTION

1. Arrangements of different chapters like that of Kent's Repertory i.e. chapters based on anatomical division with certain exceptions which are as follows -

(1) Mind	(20)Prostate gland
(2) Vertigo	
(3) Head	(21) Urethra
(4) Eye	(22) Urine
(5) Vision	(23) Male
(6) Ear	(24) Female
(7) Hearing	(25) Larynx
(8) Nose	(26) Respiration
(9) Face	(27) Cough
(10) Mouth	(28) Expectoration
(11) Teeth	(29) Chest
(12) Throat	(30) Back
(13) External Throat	(31) Extremities
(14) Stomach	(32) Sleep
(15) Abdomen	(33) Dream
(16) Rectum	(34) Chill
(17) Stool	(35) Fever
(18) Bladder	(36) Perspiration

(19) Kidney	(37) Skin
	(38) Generals

- 1st section is on Mind and the last one, Generalities.

- Discharges, e.g. stool, sweat, expectoration and urine appear as separate sections next to the anatomical region producing them.

- Certain general conditions, such as vertigo, cough, sleep, chill, and fever appear also as separate sections.

- This repertory is divided into 38 chapters; Dream being new chapter.

2. General arrangement of rubrics in each chapter are like that of Kent's Repertory which as follows-

- Under each section rubrics run in alphabetical order.

- Symptoms are divided in groups and these groups are always following each other in this same order

1. SIDES
2. TIMES
3. MODALITIES
4. EXTENSIONS
5. LOCALIZATIONS
6. (DESCRIPTIONS OF PAIN / OTHER DESCRIPTIONS)

This order of groups is repeated at each level if needed. We can expect a hierarchical structure like this at several levels.

SIDE	TIME	MODALITIES	EXTEN SION	LOCALIZA TION	DESCRIPTION OF PAIN
Time Modalities Extension	Side Modalities Extension	Side Time Modality-T/M/E Extension	Modality	Side-T/M/E Time-S Modality S/T/M-T/M/E Extension- M	At this point, if there is a chapter with a rubric pain, there is a 'description of pain'-section. The whole table can be repeated, if the corresponding symptoms exist.

Note: 'S' stands for = Side; 'T' stands for = Time; 'M' stands for = Modality; 'E' stands for = Extension.

3.   Gradation of medicines

BOLD CAPITAL	4 Marks	1st grade
Bold small	3 marks	2nd grade
Italics	2 marks	3rd grade
Ordinary roman	1 mark	4th grade

THE SOURCES

It is primarily and mainly based on the Kent's Repertory. Other sources that were added are as follows:

1.   Different authentic Repertories like Boger Boenninghausen's Characteristic Repertory, O.E. Boericke's Repertory, Phatak's Repertory and others.

2.   Different Materia Medicas of some classical authors like Hahnemann, Kent's Materia Medica, Hering's Encyclopedia, Allen's Encyclopedia, Robert's "Sensation as if ", other source books of Materia Medica e.g. Clarke's dictionary, William Boericke's Materia Medica, Phatak's Materia Medica, Tyler's Drug Picture etc.

3.   Some clinical observations from different authentic living authorities.

4.   New proving from reliable sources like Louis Klein, Jeremy Sherr and Nuala Eising etc.

NO. OF MEDICINES

Synthesis 9.1 version is the latest one and contains 2373 remedies.

SOME SPECIAL FEATURES OF SYNTHESIS

In making this repertory more authentic and more up-to-date, Dr. Schroyens formulated and added the following plans and construction.

1.   *Addition after repeated checking* – Synthesis contains repeatedly checked additions from the standard homoeopathic literature including Dr. Hahnemann, Kent, Hering, Allen, Boericke, Knerr etc. Additions from

other living authorities have been included only after proper verification.

2. *Correction of Kent's repertory* – These corrections are recognized by indicating '$_K$'. E.g. Delusion – Starve he must – Kali.chl. Is corrected to Delusion – Starve he must – Kali.m.$_{hrl,k,*}$. Here corrected source is Hering's 'Guiding symptoms of our Materia medica'. In this way thousands of corrections have been made.

3. *Symptoms are re-written in clearly readable format* – Many symptoms are rewritten in proper readable symptom format. For better comprehension at each level the words follow each other in normal order or the symptom is split with indicating sign " " to show the place from which one should start reading. Example – "pieces, sensation as if head would fall in when stooping". It is correctly written as "pieces, on stooping; sensation as if head would fall in".

4. *Combined modalities* – are applied throughout Synthesis, such as aggravation from 'cold wet weather' it would be searched as 'weather-cold-wet', but never under 'cold-damp-weather' and 'damp-cold-weather'.

5. *Clarification of ambiguous words* – Ambiguous words have been clarified wherever necessary. Example – 'breast' have been replaced by 'mammae' or 'chest' and 'storm' by 'stormy weather' or 'thunderstorm'.

6. *Creation of some rubrics* – Some more important and useful rubrics are created so that more appropriateness of the meaning of the symptoms can be achieved such as 'periodicity', 'children'.

7. *Revision of language* – correction of some nineteenth century spelling have been corrected by modern American English spelling like

- Anaemia   →   Anemia
- Diarrhoea   →   Diarrhea
- Faeces   →   Feces

8. All symptoms with 'ailments from' have been grouped in separate sub rubrics under the rubric 'ailments from'.

9. Aversion, desire, aggravation, amelioration related to food are placed under rubric *'food and drink'* in the chapter *'Generals'*.

10. *Several clinical rubrics are renamed* – Clinical conditions are renamed according to modern disease names e.g. 'hay fever' for 'coryza – annual', 'decubitus' for 'skin become sore'.

11. All dreams are present in a **separate chapter 'Dream'** following 'Sleep'.

12. *Similar rubrics are merged into one*, such as 'nose-obstruction-alternating sides' it is corrected into 'nose-obstruction-one side alternately'.

13. *Use of leading words* – Leading words have been placed in front of each level and the alphabetical sorting were corrected accordingly e.g. 'in bed' become 'bed in' and 'as if frozen' became 'frozen as if' etc.

14. *Formation of complete and clear symptoms* – Insufficiently clear symptom became much more completed on the basis of knowledge of materia medica e.g.- 'cough- sulphur fumes or vapours

sensation of agg' becomes 'cough-sulphur fumes or vapour, cough agg. by sensation of'.

15. *Use of more comprehensible words* – seldom used words have been replaced by contemporary words for better understanding e.g. 'dypsomania' became 'alcoholism'; 'childbed' became 'delivery after'.

16. *New standard list of remedy abbreviations* – A new standard list of remedy abbreviation is presented. Many new remedies have been added, all abbreviations of following the same rules used by Kent. The differences between abbreviations of Synthesis and those used so far in Kent or in Barthel's Synthetic repertory are printed in the beginning of this book. *The full list and all comments follow at the end.*

17. *New standard list of Author abbreviations* – A new standard list of author abbreviations is presented as well. Letters are used to indicate an author. This allows more combinations and easier to memorize. *No single addition has been made without indicating the source.* One reference refers to only one author, if possible even to exactly one book or article, which makes it even easier to go back to the sources. *The full list of reference is found at the end of this repertory.*

18. *Index of important changes and corrections* – All changes have been annotated with great care in order to allow verification. Thousands of references and synonyms have been incorporated where a change was made to well rubrics or remedies.

When it was not possible to indicate the change, the correction was mentioned in the *"index of important changes and corrections"* which *can be found in the end of this repertory.*

Some special features of chapter 'MIND'

- More rubric and medicines are added in the chapter mind in comparison to Kent's repertory.

- About 529 rubrics are present in Kent's repertory whereas in Synthesis it is 848.

- The following rubrics are added in Mental chapters
  Ailments from – anger
  bad news
  disappointment
  indignation etc.

- ANIMALS:
  Love for animals-
  cats:
  dogs : aeth.
  –   pet; her: med, nat-m, podo.
  children; in: med.

- NATURE: love: care. Etc.

- BEHAVIOUR Problems:
  –   children in (destructiveness, disobedience, insolence, Restlessness, rudeness etc in children.)

- BUSINESSMEN: worn – out businessmen; suited to: calc, coca, kali-p. Nux-v.

- GAMBLING:
  Passion for gambling:
  Make money to:

Some special features of 'GENERALS' chapter

- In Kent's repertory there are 245 rubrics, in generals whereas in Synthesis it is 780.

The following exclusive rubrics are there:

- FOOD & DRINKS: contains all desire, aversions, and modalities.
- Few important rubrics are listed below-

Rubrics on **pathological conditions / clinical conditions**	Acetonemia; Acidosis; Acromegaly; Adrenal failure; Agranulocytosis; Alzheimer's disease; Amoebiasis; Amyotrophic lateral sclerosis; Arteriosclerosis, Down's syndrome; Leukemia; Parkinson's disease; Poliomyelitis; Polycythemia; Reiter's Syndrome; Tuberculosis; Vericose veins etc.
Rubrics of **poisoning / abuse of**	Of Aluminium; Arsenical; Mercury; Chemotheraphy; Psychotropic drugs; Quinine; Radium theraphy; X-Ray burn etc
Rubrics on **laboratory findings**	Erythrocytes decreased; Leucocytes decreased, increased; Platelets decreased; Sperms count low etc.
Rubrics on **vaccination after**	Diphtheria; DPT; Meningitis; Neurological complaints; Prophylaxis; Rabies etc.
Rubrics on **children complaints**	Delicate; Punny; Sickly; Teenagers etc.
Rubrics on **family history** of	Asthma; Cancer; Diabetes mellitus; Eczema; Gonorrhoea; Insanity; Suicidal death; Tuberculosis etc.
Rubrics on **personal history**	Abortion; Antibiotic use of; Abscess recurrent of; Birth trauma of; Bite of animal; Gonorrhoea etc.
Rubrics on **physical makeup**	Lean people; Obesity; Emaciation etc.
Rubrics on **complexions**	Dark; Fair etc.
Rubric on **moon phases**	Full moon; New moon; Waning moon; Waxing moon etc.
Rubrics on **periodicity** like	Day – Alternate day; 4th day; 10th day; Hour; Week; Month; Year etc.

Few important rubrics with corresponding drug (s) from chapter 'Generals'

Acetonemia: carb-ac

Acromegaly: carc, *Pitu*, thyr

Adrenal failure: p-benzq

Agranulocytosis: chloram, cortico, lach, sulfa

Alzheimer's disease: alum, cordyc, hell, nux-m

Amebiasis: emetin

Aspirin, from: mag-p

Blood: affection of the- arn

Camphor: from- carb-v

Chloroform; ailments from: acet-ac, phos

Chamomile: desire for- gink-b calc-p, morb, *Nux-v*, psor, puls, *Sulph*, tub

Chronic diseases, to begin treatment: calc,

Collagen diseases: des-ac, penic, saroth, suis-chord-umb

Cryptococcosis: cryptc

Cushing's syndrome: cortico, cortiso

Disabled: congenital- syph

Down's syndrome: morg-p, pert, toxo

Dystonia; autonomic: adren, tetrac

Embolism: kali-m

Eosinophilia: brass-n-o

Family history of:anemia,measles,mumps, typhoid fever, ulcers on stomach- carc

Hypotony: atra, gels

Infectious disease: acon, bell, cortiso, echi, nat-ox-act

Iodine deficiency symptoms: calc-i, fuc, sil, spong, thyr

Lepra: accompanied by clean tongue-agar

Leukocytosis: cloth, loxo-recl, tub

Many symptoms: agar, *Carc, Tub*

Menthol: from- carb-v

Mining, ailments from: card-m, nat-ar, sulph

Myasthenia gravis: cur, cytin, gels, nat-m, pic-ac, sulph

Myopathia: alum, germ-met

Myxedema: *Ars*, cortico, dor, penic, prim-o, sulfa, *Thyr*

Ossification: arteries, of- lith

Polycythemia: cean, lach

Radium treatments, from: cadm-met, caust, rad-br

Reiter's syndrome: *Med*

Sewer-gas poisoning: anthraci, *Bapt*, phyt, pyrog, *Tub*

Shock; anaphylactic: ant-t, apis, **Carb-ac,** tetox

Silica; from overdose of: camph, **Fl-ac**, hep, merc, sulph

Sjogren's syndrome: nux-m, tub, tub-m

Tetanus: anac, anag, cocc, cortico, hyper, ip, scor- Prophylaxis: **Arn**, hell, **Hyper,** lat-m, **Led**, scor, tetox, thebin, thuj

Torpor of the left side of body: acon

X-ray burn or treatment; after: cadm-met, fl-ac

ADVANTAGES OF SYNTHESIS REPERTORY

1. This repertory is based on Kentian philosophy, so very easy to use as most of us quite acquainted with Kent's repertory through its frequent use.

2. Plan and construction is planned according to Hahnemannian schema. So, it is quite easy to search the required rubric.

3. More medicines are there in synthesis repertory than previous repertories.

4. New rubrics being added, old rubrics and their corresponding medicines are verified & upgraded where required.

5. All materials are collected from reliable sources and for every new addition references are provided. So this repertory is one among the authentic repertories.

6. Rich in cross references.

7. Method of repertorization follows the Kent's method of repertorization.

8. Constant update is going on to make this repertory perfect day by day.

9. Standard format is formed while constructing this repertory.

10. New proving is being incorporated.

11. New rubrics are created as in chapter of 'Generals'- rubrics on different **pathological conditions, poisoning, complexions, children complaints, physical makeup,** vaccination after, **laboratory findings** etc. These rubrics are of immense value in present day practice and they are the gems of this repertory.

12. Rubrics on **moon phases, periodicity, family history, personal history** are the unique creation of this repertory.

SUITABILITY/ADAPTABILITY OF THE SYNTHESIS REPERTORY

Any case rich in generals and characteristic particular can be repertorized by Synthesis. A case having only characteristic particular too can be repertorized by using this repertory. Now it is so elaborated in each chapter any type of totality can be worked out with this repertory.

MERITS OF NEW REPERTORIES

We mostly depend upon Kent, BTPB, BBCR as we are all conversant with these books through their frequent use and also they have strong philosophical background. These new repertories mention about the sources from where they have been taken. In contrary, Kent has taken much information from different sources in his repertory, but he did not mention anything about the source. He even had not considered many works which remain untouched. These new repertories are of immense value and have done great benefit to the profession. Synthesis Repertory is one among the modern repertories. New rubrics being added, old rubrics and their corresponding medicines are verified & upgraded where required. New medicines are added.

LIMITATIONS

So far no drawbacks as this repertory is constantly being updating and correcting the materials except about the reliability of new additions of living authors.

B. COMPLETE REPERTORY

Author: **Dr. Roger Van Zandvoort.** Complete repertory is one of the widely used repertories since the last decade. This project work is done by the Institute of Research in Homoeopathic Information and Symptamatology.

In practice, they first treated most people with herbal medicines, but when they felt that they really knew the correct homoeopathic remedy, only when it was clear, they gave homoeopathic remedy. But after a while the entire practice was homoeopathy. And then he bought a computer in 1987, and a Mac repertory to help in practice.

Roger started comparing the information that Bill Gray had with the Vithoulkas additions to the Synthetic Repertory, and saw that there were many differences. He liked the Synthetic repertory, so he started collecting material to add to Mac Repertory and saw that the authors were not always the same, although they had the same additions. So he got involved in finding out where these additions really came from. There's a lot of information missing in Kent's Repertory, and that is one of the reasons that he began this work.

Number of drugs : 2171 approx

Book edition published : 1996

Gradation:
- First grade   : Roman
- Second grade   : *Bold – Italics*
- Third grade   : **BOLD UPPERCASE**
- Fourth grade   : **BOLD UPPERCASE AND UNDERLINED**

Some gradations were changed referring to Kent's lectures, Lesser Writings, and Minor Writings.

Philosophical background: General to Particular as that of Kent's Repertory.

Plan and construction:
The Repertory is available in the print form and electronic form. In the print form it is available as a single all in one volume or in three volumes. In the electronic form it is available with Mac Repertory / Hompath Classic / Cara etc.

The complete Repertory : Mind (Vol. I)

The complete Repertory : Vertigo to peech and voice (Vol. II)

The complete Repertory : Respiration to Generalities (Vol. III)

The basic information used to create this repertory came from the first, third and sixth American edition of Kent's Repertory.

This information was combined with many corrections and additions by checking and re-checking was found in: Homoeopathic journals.

The Complete against Kent's Repertory, Kunzli's Repertorium Generale and Schmidt's and Chand's Final General Repertory using the original sources.

- Sivaraman's Additional and corrections to Kent's Repertory
- CCRH's corrections to Boenninghausen's Repertory

- Boger's and Phatak's additions, Boenninghausen's Repertory and Boenninghausen's unique private additions.
- Boericke's Repertory additions.

In addition to these, confusing remedy abbreviations were extensively verified and corrected.

Textural changes to Kent's Repertory

1. The format of each rubric is carefully examined and inconsistencies corrected.

2. The most important word in a rubric is moved to the beginning of that rubric.

3. The rubrics were re-alphabetized.

4. The hierarchy of the rubrics is reconstructed to follow the format: General, sides (left, right), times, agg. and amel. and concordances, extending to, localizations and sensations (pain).

5. Older terminology is replaced when clearly needed by more modern terminology following the American English spelling.

6. The language of rubrics were corrected to more precisely match its materia medica source.

7. The inconsistent use of several words was replaced with the same meaning by a single word throughout.

8. The remedy abbreviations were again examined. Different abbreviations for one and the same remedy were put together.

9. The remedies in each rubric were re-alphabetized, according to the alphabetical order of the abbreviations instead of the alphabetical order of the full names of the remedies.

Reorganizing rubrics:

There have been some important changes to some of the main rubrics in the mind section. The dreams have been put in the mind section. After speaking to many homoeopaths the general idea has formed that the dreams are a substantial part of the mind section. The dreams represent emotional impressions and mental strain.

The location of the main rubrics and their sub rubrics for Speech in the Mind and Mouth section of the Repertory has changed.

The original reason that Kent used Speech in the Mind section and another part of speech in the mouth section, was that he wanted to make a difference for those sub rubrics of speech, that had a mental – emotional aetiology, as distinct from those sub rubrics of speech, that were more patho-physiological in their aetiology. Nevertheless, many rubrics have seen confused or were open to mis-interpretation. What it is done is the meaning of the rubrics was reexamined and then used them in the new chapter for speech and voice, it was used them under other main rubrics, mainly talk, talking, talks, when the aetiology was more of emotional – mental one.

The main rubric speech under speech and voice includes all those rubrics that are more connected to the motor control of speech.

The separate rubrics talk, talking and talks have been combined into one rubric named talk, talking, talks since they were inconsistent in their meaning and therefore confusing.

The bodily anxieties and apprehensions have been included in the mind section under anxiety. The reason for this is that, although felt in a specific part of the body, it is still an expression of emotional value and therefore should be included in the mind section. Of course we also preserved those rubrics in the specific body part section.

The sub rubrics dealing with animals and body or body parts under the main rubrics delusions, dreams and fear have been collected together in large sun rubrics.

In delusions many sub rubrics with the same meaning were found and their remedies were transferred to the most likely place to find that information. Cross-references were inserted, where the rubric had been in the Kent's Repertory, to indicate t where it has been moved.

All of those moves can be traced by using the search mechanism to find all occurrences of any word and its synonyms.

In all chapters the Discolorations and Eruptions have been re-organized so that all of their sub rubrics now have the same hierarchical layout.

All the pains, except for the Head pain section and Extremity pain section, have been reorganized hierarchically. They all start with General, followed by the time modalities, the general modalities and causations, the "extending to" rubrics followed by the pain types, including 'wandering", "radiating" and "pulsating/throbbing".

Additions

Additions were made from various sources, using information about the reliability of authors, and using the book reviews for those sources from old homoeopathic journals as a guideline for quality.

As a general rule, additions were made from the oldest author available for that addition. The grade of the additions and the existing information were also taken into account, in order not to destroy the valid information in Kent's Repertory.

The original source is credited with their additions. In most cases there is extensive materia medica available to confirm and check information.

New rubrics

New rubrics were created when there were no existing rubrics that covered their Materia Medica meaning in Kent's Repertory. The meaning of the rubric was studied using the information in the materia medica and the information in contemporary dictionaries, from the time that the information become available. Also, the rubric to be added should have real homoeopathic value, i.e. the new information should be information that helps the consulting homoeopaths find the right remedy.

Cross-references

To help locate as many close alternatives to a specific rubric as possible, most of the similar, but still somewhat different rubrics have been included as cross-references for many rubrics. This gives us better choices for our patients.

References and cross-references

References are connected to rubrics that have no remedies and points to the rubrics to look at that certain remedies. References start with a " ' " sign, followed by a " . " for every next reference.

Cross references are connected to rubrics that have remedies and will follow behind the remedies of that rubric pointing to the rubrics with related meanings. Cross references always start with a . sign.

References can be found in the same main rubric or sub rubric, depending on the location of the rubric these references are referring to, when these first references are written in lower case italics.

If the reference is pointing to a main rubric then the first letter of that rubric as a reference is displayed in upper case italic and the other characters in lower case italics.

If the reference indicating another section of the Repertory then that sections name in the reference is displayed in upper case italic.

Author identification numbers

The author identification numbers (ID's) are based on chronology, based on the dates that the listed authors first published their work. This is a change from the system used in the pre – 3.1 computer versions of the Complete Repertory, the Synthetic Repertory and the Repertorium Generale. The new system enables to have an idea about the time the addition has been made and by whom. Author numbers are displayed as subscript numbers behind the remedy abbreviation.

The last three numbers of an author number are used to specify the authors place in the chronological system we used that starts with the 1 for Hahnemann S. as being the oldest homoeopath to, at this point in the development of the Complete Repertory, 239 Riefer M. as the last person added to the list and therefore the most recent author that we took additions or new remedy names from. Since this work started with a rather complete list of authors, while giving everyone a suitable ID number, most ID numbers fall into the 3 digit category. Nevertheless and of course, some authors have been added later in the process. These authors got 4 digit numbers where the first digit only indicates the first, second, third or even fourth time of renumbering.

Therefore

- Hahnemann S.
- Stapf E.
- 1002 Hartmann F. (from the same time as Stapf, but added in the first re-numbering session).
- 2002 Jorg J.C.G. (from the same time as Stapf, but added in the second re-numbering session)
- 100 Blackwood A.L
- 1100 Shedd P.W (from the same time as Blackwood, but added in the first re-numbering session).

Repertory page references

Page references for Kent's Repertory [K], the Synthetic Repertory [SI, SII or SIII] and the Repertorium Generale [G] have been included for those rubrics that are mentioned in these repertories directly behind the rubric text.

Enhancing main rubrics

In the Complete repertory main rubrics always include in the remedies found in their sub rubrics. From the view point that e repertory is first of all an index to the material medica that policy can easily be redefended. All remedies in sub rubrics not in the main rubric have been added in plain type. When the remedy was already in the main rubric by a later author (often Kent) then the author for that remedy in the sub rubric the remedy in the main rubric got the author in the sub rubric. The grade of that remedy in the main rubric was kept as it was. Depending on the way one repertories this can be very useful and in cases where patients cannot be specific enough about their symptoms it is more than welcome to have a complete collection of all possible remedies in the main rubric. The enhancement should not make homoeopaths use main rubrics only. Homoeopathically, it is still the best to go the most specific (sub) rubric in order to find the similimum, if possible.

Remedy abbreviations

Some remedy abbreviations have been changed to ensure that there will be less confusion about what each abbreviation denotes. The confusion was particularly marked for the mineral salts, acidums and aceticum. Also where some remedies have been known by more than one Latin abbreviation this has been corrected.

Special features

- Certainty about finding the correct rubrics and remedies

- A complete overview of related rubrics using cross – references

- A choice of information from old and new sources, using the latest provings.

- The best possibilities curing your patients

- And it is the most comprehensive repertory in existence because it has: more than 515,000 checked additions.

C. MURPHYS REPERTORY

ABOUT AUTHOR:

Dr. Robin Murphy was born on August 15, 1950 in Grand Rapids, Michigan, USA to Calvin & Verna Murphy.

- He carried out his undergraduate studies at the Michigan State University.(1972-1976).
- There he discovered their homoeopathic historical collection and became intrigued with the system and began his studies.
- Robin Murphy has a great interest in medical alchemy, the Egyptian medicine.
- He finds Hahnemann's work having a great similarity with Paracelsus' work as well as Egyptian medicine.
- He has tried to correlate the three philosophical principles of Paracelsus - Sulphur, Mercury and Salt with Psora, Syphilis and Sycosis, the miasmatic theory of Hahnemann.
- Not only that he also believes that the doctrine of vital force is taken from Archeus principles of Egyptian medicine. He states, "The root of homeopathy was alchemy and that came from Egypt.
- Since homoeopathy is included in the course and curriculum of Naturopathic Medicine in America, he studied naturopathic system of medicine and got the degree of N.D. (Naturopathic Doctor). In the beginning, his prescriptions were based on Boericke and Clarke's manuals.

Later on he became fond of the Kentian School and practiced classical homoeopathy for a long time.

- Having gone through the experience of various types of prescribing in homoeopathy, he finally learned prescribing for diseases still doing classical at some time.
- Robin Murphy had his first love for history of medicine.
- In America (1970-71) while going through the various medical literatures he came across some homeopathic journals from 1800's, which were lying idle.
- He was shocked to see the plethora of literature available on homeopathy.
- As he went through them he developed more and more interest in the system.
- Initially he learned homoeopathy on his own from the study of journals, books and various case materials, later he wanted to do a regular course in homoeopathy.
- Robin Murphy is one of the best known teachers of homeopathy in the world.
- He has extensive teaching and clinical experience including his years as chairman of the homoeopathic department at the National College of Naturopathic medicine in Portland.
- He has lectured at the national center for homoeopathy and at colleges in Canada and England.
- He is now director of the Hahnemann academy of North America.
- His repertory and Materia Medica are now standard texts in colleges throughout the world.

- As we understood the most widely accepted Repertory in twentieth century have been Kent Repertory.

- Murphy repertory has undergone a step more in the indexing of the symptoms of materia medica & rearranging it in the alphabetical way. So an enthusiastic student & learner of homoeopathy cannot keep away from this valuable repertory

- Dr. Robin Murphy is known worldwide for his published works. He authored the Homoeopathic Medical Repertory in 1993 and the Lotus Materia Medica in 1996. Both the works have been well appreciated by the homoeopathic fraternity.

- In modern terms the Homeopathic Medical Repertory represents experimental and therapeutic database for the practice of homeopathic medicine.

- The general information contained in the homeopathic repertories and Materia Medicas are derived from the following sources history, provings, clinical practice, research, physiology and toxicology.

- The Homeopathic Medical Repertory was designed to be a model practical and easy to use clinical guide to the vast homeopathic Materia Medica.

- To achieve these goals a completely new repertory had to be constructed with a new schema, terminology, chapters, clinical rubric additions and upgrades.

- Also there was a great need to fill in the clinical deficiencies and to correct the major flaws found in the older repertories.

- After prolonged research and experimentation with the old schemas, he decided to create a new one that would facilitate access to rubrics at all levels and to provide clearer images of the anatomical, physiological and clinical rubric groups.

- Now, all the lungs rubrics are in one place, instead of being spread throughout the chest chapter. This allows easy jumping from particular to general chapters or the other way around.

- If one cannot find a pain rubric in it's precise location (lungs), then go to the more general rubrics of the chest chapter. Be aware that the chest pain rubrics are more general and include heart pain also.

- The first edition of this book was published in1993. First Indian edition came in May 1994, published by IBPS New Delhi. This book has been dedicated to DR.KIRPAL SINGH.

- The second edition was published in the year 1996. This was published with new addition and Indian Books & Periodicals Publishers, New Delhi, published Indian edition in October 2002. In this three more chapters were added and they are constitution, disease and headache. First reprint edition came in 2004.

- All of Kent's repertory & sections of Knerr's Repertory were used as the foundation for building this new repertory.

- 55 major sources of addition are given in first edition.

- In first edition this was given before repertory proper.

- In second edition it is given after repertory proper.
- As per alphabetical order of authors name books are arranged.
- 56 books are given in second edition. Added source in this edition is Witco D. C.A.R.A.

Homeopathic References Major Sources of Additions and New Rubrics:

- Allen, H. C., Keynotes and Characteristics, Mat. Med. Of the Nosodes, Therapeutics of Fever.
- Allen, J. H., Diseases and Therapeutics of the Skin.
- Allen, T. F., Encyclopedia of Pure Mat. Med., Handbook of Mat. Med. And Homeopathic Therapeutics, Symptom-Register.
- Anschutz E. P., New, Old and Forgotten Remedies.
- Barthel H., and Klunker, W., The Synthetic Repertory.
- Bell J. B., Therapeutics of Diarrhea.
- Boenninghausen, C.M. and Boger, C.M., Characteristics and Repertory, Therapeutic Pocket Book.
- Boericke, Wm. and O. E., Manual of Horn. Mat. Med. and Repertory.
- Boger, C. M., A Synoptic key of the Materia Medica, Additions to Kent's Repertory, Moon Phases, Times of Remedies.
- Borland, D. M., Children's Types, Homeopathic Practice.

11. Burnett, J. C., Fifty Reasons for being a Homeopath, Organ Diseases of Women, Diseases of the Liver and Spleen, Vaccinosis.

12. Clarke, J. H., Clinical Repertory, Dictionary of Practical Mat. Med., Prescriber.

13. Dewey, W. A., Essentials of Horn eo. Mat. Med., Practical Homeopathic Therapeutics, 12 Tissue Remedies.

14. Eizayaga, F. X., EI Moderno Repertorio de Kent.

15. Farrington, E. A., Clinical Materia Medica, Comparative Materia Medica.

16. Foubister, D., Carcinosin Research, Tutorials on Homeopathy.

17. Gallavardin, J., Repertory of Psychic Medicines & Materia Medica.

18. Gentry, W. D., The Concordance Repertory.

19. Gibson, D., Studies of Homeopathic Remedies.

20. Guernsey, H. N., Keynotes to the Materia Medica, Obstetrics.

21. Gupta, B. P., Encyclopedia of Homeopathy.

22. Hahnemann, S., Materia Medica Pura and Chronic Diseases.

23. Hale, E. M., Homeo.Mat. Med. of New Remedies, Diseases of the Heart.

24. Hansen, 0., Textbook of Mat. Med. and Therapeutics of Rare Remedies.

25. Hering, C., Analytical Repertory of Symptoms of the Mind, The Guiding Symptoms of our Mat. Med.

26. Hughes, R. & Dake, J. P., A Cyclopaedia of Drug Pathogenesy.

27. Imhauser, H., Homeopathy in Pediatric Practice.

28. Jahr, G. H. G., A New Manual of Homeopathic Practice.

29. Julian, O. A, Mat. Med. of New Homeo. Remedies, Diet. of Mat. Med.

30. Kent, J. T., Repertory of the Materia Medica, (as well as his handwritten corrections of the last American edition of the Repertory), Lectures on Homeopathic Materia Medica, Lesser Writings, New Remedies.

31. Kichlu and Bose, A Textbook of Descriptive Medicine.

32. Knerr, C. A, Repertory of Herings Guiding Symptoms of our Mat. Med.

33. Kunzli, J., Kent's Repertorium Generale.

34. Lathoud, J. A., Homeopathic Materia Medica.

35. Lilienthal, S., Homeopathic Therapeutics.

36. Lippe, C., Repertory to the Characteristic Symptoms of the Mat. Med.

37. Minton H., Uterine Therapeutics.

38. Murphy, R., Lotus Materia Medica, Lectures on Homeopathic Medi-cines, Homeopathic Philosophy & Practice, Medical Alchemy, Lotus Medical Library, Audio Lecture Series, on cassette tapes).

39. Nash, E. B., Leaders in Homeopathic Therapeutics.

40. Patel, R. P., Word Index with Rubrics of Kent's Repertory.

41. Phatak, S. R., Concise Repertory of Homeopathic Remedies, Materia Medica of Homeopathic Remedies.

42. Roberts, H. A, Sensations as if, Studies of Remedies by Comparison.

43. Royal, G., Textbook of Homeopathic Materia Medica.

44. Schussler,W., The Biochemic System, The Twelve Tissue Remedies.

45. Sirker, C., A Keynote Repertory of Materia Medica.

46. Sheppard, D., Epidemic Diseases, Magic of the Minimum Dose.

47. Stephenson, J., A Mat. Med. and Repertory, Hahnemannian Provings.

48. Tyler, M. L., Homeo. Drug Pictures, Pointers to Common Remedies.

49. Underwood B. F., The Diseases of Childhood and Their Homeopathic Treatment, Headaches and Its Materia Medica.

50. Van Zandvoort., The Complete Repertory. (Computer Repertory)

51. Von Lippe, A, Keynotes and Redline Symptoms ofthe Materia Medica.

52. Vithoulkas, G., Additions to Kent's Repertory.

53. Ward, J. W., Unabridged Dictionary of the Sensations As If.

54. Warkentin, D. K., MacRepertory, ReferenceWorks, (Computer)

55. Witko, D., CAR.A, (Computer)

56. Yingling, W. A, The Accoucheurs Emergency Manual.
   • Using the modern terminology is paramount to the study and practice of homeopathy.
   • The language of the provings, Materia Medicas, therapeutic books and in the repertories must reflect the culture one lives in.

- If the homeopathic provings and the case taking protocols require us to record a person's symptoms in their own words, shouldn't the repertory have a similar language?

- The formatting for the Homeopathic Medical Repertory is similar to Kent's Repertory with the strongest remedies in the rubric or sub-rubric are designated in bold-capitals, CARC., (3 points), next, bold-italics, care., (2 points) and plain-type, carc., (1 point).

- In general, if a remedy has cured a symptom or condition more than three times and it's been confirmed by more than three homeopaths it deserves to be added to the repertory in the lowest grade, (1 point, plain type).

- If a remedy has cured more than six times and likewise confirmed by three others, it should be added in the second grade, (2 points, bold-italics).

- The third grade (3 points, bold-capital) requires twelve cases plus confirmations by three or more practitioners.

- The editing of the manuscript was then done which involved adding modern terminology, cross references and correcting errors.

- The final step was to systematically survey the homeopathic literature for reliable additions to add to the alphabetical repertory.

- The highest Priority was to find clinical information relevant to modern homeopathic practice and to fill in the areas where Kent's

Repertory is weak in information. (Mental disorders, emergencies, infections, pathologies and major organs).

- The result is the Homeopathic Medical Repertory, which contains 70 chapters, consistent formatting, (alphabetical chapters, rubrics and sub-rubrics), modern terminology, and modern diseases, with 40,000 new rubrics, 200,000 new additions and updates, in a small lightweight size for convenience.

- The second edition of the Homeopathic Medical Repertory was written to be a major upgrade of the first edition.

- All the column headers and the word index entries were completely re-done, expanded and corrected.

- The word index was also expanded to include many more clinical conditions and states.

- The Homeopathic Remedies list was moved to the front of the book for easier access to the names abbreviations of all the homoeopathic and herbal remedies.

- The Homeopathic References list was moved to the back of the book.

- The vast majority of the new additions came from hering Guiding Symptoms and Allens Symptoms Index of the Encyclopedia of Pure Materia Medica. Jeremy Sherr's provings and clinical observations on the homeopathic uses of Chocolate, (Choco.), Hydrogen, (Hydrog.) and Scorpion, (Scorp) are included in this edition.

- The Homeopathic Medical Repertory now has 70 chapters. Three new chapters were created from the original 67 chapters found in the first edition. These are: Diseases, Constitutions and Headaches.

- The new Disease chapter contains all the pathological and tissue rubrics from the Generals chapter plus the primary disease and inflammation rubrics from other chapters.

- The Disease chapter contains: diseases, disorders, ailments, degenerative states, tissue changes, abscesses, allergies, atrophy, cancers, convalescence, edema, emaciation, growths, herpes, infections, inflammations, miasms, organs, suppressions, tumors.

- The new Constitutions chapter contains all the genetic, dispositions and body types from the Generals chapter.

- Extensive additions were gathered from Hering's Guiding Symptoms.

- The Constitutions chapter contains: constitutions, temperaments, body size, body type, hair in general, complexions, age, growth, gender, habits, defects, miasms, infants, inheritance, children, boys, girls, elderly people, men, occupations, women, young people.

- The Headaches chapter was created out of the Head chapter.

- The new Headaches chapter contains all the head pain rubrics, types of pain, causative factors, concomitants, modalities, times of day, seasons, locations, head general, forehead, occiput, sides, temples, vertex.

- The Generals chapter was rewritten, the pain and sensation rubrics are now found in alphabetical order instead of being sub-rubrics in the pain and sensations sections. This matches the alphabetical format of all the other chapters of the repertory.

- All the chapters of the Homeopathic Medical Repertory have been re-examined, corrected and updated with clinical additions.

- New page numbers are due to the new chapters, additions and formatting.

- The Homeopathic Medical Repertory and the Lotus Materia Medica are also available on computer programs for the Macintosh and IBM formats. These programs are available from:

- Kent Homeopathic Associates, 710 Mission Avenue, San Rafael, California, U.S.A., 94901, (Mac Repertory & Reference Works)

- Miccant Software, 14 Mulberry Close, West Bridgford, Nottingham, United Kingdom, NG2-7SS, (C.A.R.A & Similia)

- Located in the front pages of the Medical Repertory.

- Includes the abbreviations used in the Homeopathic Medical Repertory and the Lotus Materia Medica, plus the full Latin names and common names for many homoeopathic and herbal remedies."

- Each drug is alphabetically arranged as per drug abbreviation, given in roman letters both the genus and species. Continued by full Latin names & their common names.
- Each alphabet is mentioned under that drugs of that alphabet are mentioned.
- If it is cross-referenced to another drug, it is given with = sign.
- If it is a cross reference of a drug then it is given in brackets with= sign. Even certain cross-references are given in brackets. e.g. ether, dolichos, etc. certain places words found in brackets are not cross references, these may be synonyms. E.g. bry, chin, iris tenax. Total 27 pages.
- HIERARCHICAL-Anatomical-Boenninghausen, Boericke, Lippe, Kent, Knerr.
- CONCORDANCE-Symptomatic - Allen, Clark, Gentry, Phatak.
- ALPHABETICAL-Clinical-Murphy.
- Historically, Hahnemann first constructed an outline for recording the information gathered from the experimental provings of the homeopathic remedies. This eventually became the schema for his Materia Medica Pura.
- In Hahnemann's preface to his Materia Medica Pura he gives the complete layout on pages 4-5.
- Kent's Repertory is based on the assumption that all cases should be analyzed from the generals to the particulars. Kent saw his cases from one perspective only; therefore he was a prejudiced observer even before he took a case!
- It is a common myth in modern homeopathy that mental symptoms are more important than physical ones. The particular symptoms coming from tumors, diseased organs or wounds can literary kill a person, which makes local symptoms the most important in many cases.
- A natural hierarchy used for case analysis has to be based on what life treating to the patient, next, the causative factors in the case and then, the most severe or important presenting symptoms.
- In case analysis there never was a fixed hierarchy in the homeopathic literature and there never will be because it goes against the individualization of each natural hierarchy in a healthy person is physiological, in a sick person that natural order becomes deranged into multiple unpredictable patterns.
- We are not suppose to have preconceived ideas about what should be important in a case, we should perceive the unique hierarchy of every case.
- Thus it is an alphabetical general clinical book form repertory.
- There are 1851 drugs.
- BOLD CAPITALS bold italics roman type
- 3 marks 2 marks 1 mark

- The Alphabetical Format
- For the new repertory, 70 chapters were created and rearranged in an alphabetical order from the original 36 chapters found in Kent's Repertory.
- The Homeopathic Medical Repertory was created to be more consistent with Hahnemann's anatomical and physiological categories reorganized into an alphabetical order. The alphabetical format was chosen as the most natural method to organize large amounts of information, thus bringing the repertory in line with all the large homeopathic materia medicas, which are also alphabetically arranged.
- All of the chapters are arranged alphabetically according to anatomy, physiology or clinical topic.
- All the rubrics and sub rubrics within each chapter were also sorted into an alphabetical schema. Thereby simplifying Kent's complicated system for arranging rubrics and sub rubrics, by sides, time, conditions, modalities, circumstances, extensions, locations, etc.
- In second edition three more chapters were added and they are constitution, disease and headache.
- The editing of the manuscript was then done which involved adding modern terminology, cross references and correcting errors.
- The final step was to systematically survey the homeopathic literature for reliable additions to add to the alphabetical repertory.
- While forming this repertory the highest priority is given to find clinical information relevant to modern homoeopathic practice and to fill in the areas where Kent repertory is weak in information (e.g. Mental disorders, emergencies, infections, pathologies and major organs).
- There is complete reorganization of the information with small anatomical and functional subdivisions in alphabetical order.
- Resulting this repertory; contains thirty new chapters, consistent formatting (alphabetical chapters, rubrics sub rubrics), and modern disorder with 40,000 new rubrics, 200000 new additions and updates in a small lightweight size for convenience.
- There is bold reorganization and expansion of repertorial information with many practical divisions such as with children, pregnancy, emergences, the environment, dreams and delusions, including use of modern diagnostic terminology as Alzheimer's syndrome, Disc syndrome, Polycystic ovaries etc.
- The abbreviations used are agg. = aggravates, worse from or symptoms increased by. amel. = ameliorates, better from or symptoms decreased by.
- Each chapter starts in a fresh page.
- The chapter name given in bold roman in top right side of page in right page & left side of left page. Similarly page number given.

- Chapter number given only in starting page.

  Then chapter name is given in italics in beginning page under which rubrics and sub rubrics are mentioned. Each page is divided into double column for easy view & space convenience.

  The chapters as well as the rubrics are arranged alphabetically. Parts of the chapter 'Extremities' itself constitute 12 chapters in Murphy's Repertory. They are Shoulders Hip Arms Legs Elbow Knee Wrist Ankle Hand Feet Limbs & Joints.

  The most important among the new chapters are: 1. Children. 2. Emergency. 3. Environment. 4. Glands. 5. Intestines. 6. Joints.7. Neck. 8. Nerves.9. Pregnancy. & 10. Toxicity.

- Others are Blood,Bones, Brain, Delusions, Dreams, Food, Heart, Knees, Liver, Lungs, Muscles, Pelvis, Pulse, Tongue, etc.

- Mind chapter is the biggest chapter with 161 pages. Next biggest is Headache with 89 pages..

- Smallest chapter: Elbow with 6 pages & 66 rubrics, wrist with 6 pages & 64 rubrics.

- The generals contain a bigger group of medicines followed by sub rubrics, which are arranged alphabetically. Therefore, alphabetical arrangement is the only principle followed in this repertory.

- Though the foundation of constructing this new repertory is based on Repertory of the Homoeopathic' Materia Medica by Dr. J. T. Kent, it does not follow the arrangement of side, time or modalities and extensions.

- Main rubrics – bold capital

- Sub rubric - ordinary roman, found 2 indentations inner to main rubric, followed by '-' drugs given alphabetically in its typography.

- Sub sub rubric – ordinary roman, found 2 indentations inner to sub rubric, followed by '-' drugs given alphabetically in its typography.

- Mostly under locations main rubric is repeated in roman bold, 2 indentations inner to main rubric.

- In few places main rubric is repeated in bold capital. E.g. page 15, especially describing particular locations.

- Main rubric repeated. E.g. DELUSIONS, PEOPLE, STRANGERS, COUGHING, PERIODIC

- In few places sub rubrics given in bold roman. E.g. Menses, page 40, 217 especially for discharge, pain, expressions, etc.

- Rubrics if continues in second column given in capitals. E.g. page 352, 353.

- Before during, after given as during given directly with main rubric. before & after as alphabetically. E.g. page 880, page 923, Eating, page 159, burning, urination.

- In Head locations given alphabetically.

- Extending to, rubrics given alphabetically. E.g. page 909

- Female leucorrhoea (See Discharge vagina),
- Here urethra given in Bladder chapter.
- Cross-references are of 2 types:
- Cross-reference with drugs e.g. page No: 1 Abscess (See Buboes), Aching pain (See Pain Abdomen)
- Cross-reference without drugs e.g. page 21, Dropsy, (See Ascites)
- Cross reference given in ordinary roman.
- Like Knerr the sections are made as chapters in many places. Mostly in provers language.
- Biggest rubric COUGH, Croupy.
- Kent said in his repertory's preface, "Physicians are requested to send in verified and clinical symptoms, and to call attention to any errors which they may discover in the text. " Referring to how the repertory was compiled he admits the rubrics came from two major sources the materia medica and notes from our ablest practitioners, these notes are the clinical rubrics, upgrades and additions when verified in homeopathic practice.
- Hahnemann states throughout the Organon, that every homeopath must clearly perceive what has to be cured in diseases, and to perceive the totality of symptoms of the disease. He also refers to acute diseases, chronic diseases, epidemic diseases, iatrogenic diseases, infectious dis-eases, mental diseases, miasmatic diseases, physical diseases, traumatic diseases, etc.
- Therefore, homeopathic repertories must include more clinical rubrics, especially ones that reflect the new diseases and conditions of our modern chemical-industrial society and those cause by allopathic drugs, radiation, chemotherapy, surgery, vaccinations, etc. (see the Diseases, Emergency, Fevers and Toxicity chapters).
- The Homeopathic Medical Repertory is based on the principles of clinical as well as classical homeopathic practice.
- This repertory merges both kinds of practice unlike many other repertories and it has the advantage of meeting the requirement of various types of cases.
- The author's aim to make it a modern, practical and easy reference book has enriched this repertory with many clinical as well as pathological rubrics.
- The chapters on Environment, Generals, Food, Mind, Perspiration, Constitution, Dreams, Delusion, etc. help us to go through more classical generals to particulars whereas chapters like Disease, Emergency, Children, Toxicity, Blood, etc. contain plenty of clinical rubrics.
- This is a unique repertory, which help practitioner to find out the similimum on the basis of clinical as well as classical symptoms.
- The author has merged both the types of practice, i.e. classical and clinical. He says, "If you do only

one type, you are a half homeopath.

- Learn to prescribe according to the case." He further states "The right way to prescribe is revealed in the case and by the results that you get, not by some old theory and principles.
- Located at the end of the Medical Repertory.
- Given with a representation of each alphabet.
- Chapter words given in bold roman.
- Each word is given with page numbers given in 3 columns for space convenience.
- This list is used to find particular words and clinical references such as influenza or hepatitis.
- Common words found in most chapters such as burning, are not included in the Word Index because they are easily accessible alphabetically within each chapter, (Headaches, throbbing).
- Murphy's concept of totality is based on clinical as well as classical homeopathic practice.
- It embraces the principles of Kent's generals, Boenninghausen's complete symptoms, Boger's pathological generals and other stalwarts' clinical principles of prescribing.
- He believes in constructing the totality as per the details available in the case.
- If the case has more generals Kent's principles should be followed for erecting a totality.

- If the case has complete symptoms, rich concomitants and pathological generals Boenninghausen's and Boqer's principles should be followed.
- Murphy feels that there are many opinions in homeopathy, which is not healthy.
- A practical man, who believes in results and not mere theories, has a strong conviction in the law of similar.
- Being disgusted with various opinions he says, "Homeopathy is probably the most opinionated medical science on the whole planet where groups with opinions and theories feel that they have the answer to Homeopathy.
- This repertory can be used for all types of cases:
- Where the case, has a paucity of symptoms.
- Where generals are prominent
- Where clinical symptoms / diagnosis is available
- Pathological generals/ constitutions are available
- Where complete symptoms are available.
- All types of cases can be worked by using Homeopathic Medical Repertory.
- The following methods can be applied de-pending upon the data available in the case:
- Generals to particulars
- Complete symptom
- Pathological Generals
- Causation

- Concomitant
- Clinical rubrics
- Modalities.
- If we compare three rubrics of Murphy repertory with that of complete repertory of Mac Repertory - Deceitful, Defiant & Ailments from reproaches.
- In Deceitful - Lyco(2), opium(3) and thuja are upgraded in Murphy repertory. When compared with the complete repertory and Morphinum is added.
- In defiant - Cham(2) and Medo(1) are added and Tuber is upgraded to (3) marks.
- In ailments from reproaches Dr. Murphy has added Anac(1), Cham~1), lyco(3) -Nat. Mur(2) and upgraded carcinoma(2), Colocy(2) and staphysagria(3).
- In many rubrics where single drug is mentioned under Kent repertory, in Murphy repertory more number of drugs is mentioned which provides a vast magnitude and scope to the Homoeopathic Physician, but again controversy arises about their sources.
- For example:
- Itching with jaundice - Hepar sulph(1) (KR)
- Itching with jaundice - Dolichos, Hepar sulph(2),Myrica(1),Pic acid, Ran bulb, thy, trinit.
- Hairs, unusual part on - Thuj (KR)
- Hairs, unusual part on - Carci, Lyco, Medo, Thuj, Tub.
- Missing chapters when compared to Kent's repertory:
- Expectoration, Urethra, Prostate gland.
- Important variations in subsections of chapters when compared to Kent's Repertory:
- Axilla is seen under Shoulder chapter. (Under Chest in Kent.)
- Expectoration is seen under lungs chapter. (As a separate chapter in Kent.)
- Urethra is seen under Bladder chapter. (As a separate chapter in Kent.)
- Prostate gland under Male chapter. (As a separate chapter in Kent.)
- Oesophagus under Stomach chapter. (Under Throat in Kent)
- Lips under Mouth chapter. (Under Face in Kent)
- . Hair under Generalities. (Under different chapters-Head, face etc., in Kent)
- Nates under Pelvis. (Under extremities in Kent)
- Convulsions under Nerves. (Under Generalities in Kent.)
- Seasonal modalities in Environment. (Under Generalities in Kent)
- Palpitation in Heart. (Under Chest in Kent)
- Coccyx & Sacrum in Pelvis (under back in Kent)
- Perineum in Pelvis. (Under rectum in Kent)
- Thyroid in Glands. (Under throat in Kent)
- Noises in Hearing. (Under ear in Kent)

- **Important variations in terms used when compared to Kent's Repertory:**
  - Murphy * Kent.
  - Discharge, Vaginal * Leucorrhoea.
  - Epistaxis * Nosebleeds
  - Insomnia * Sleeplessness
  - Hemorrhages * Bleeding
  - Headache * Pain (Head chapter)
  - Appetite, loss of * Appetite, wanting
  - Belching * Eructation
  - Legs * Lower limbs
  - Miscarriage * Abortion

- **Examples for Rubrics, which are not available in Kent's Repertory:**
  - Fevers, Rheumatic Fever.
  - Throat, Adenoids.
  - Nose, Sinusitis, headache from sinus catarrh.
  - Lungs, asthma, Heart problems with.
  - Stomach, pain, Vomiting, amel

1. This repertory has more than 39,000 new rubrics and 2,00,000 new additions and updates.

2. It contains all valuable information from standard homeopathic literatures and repertories.

3. It has a total of 70 chapters alphabetically arranged. The new charters like Children, Emergencies, Toxicity etc. are very helpful to professionals. There are new chapters on major organs like Liver, Lung, Heart, etc.

4. Many clinical rubrics are added to each chapter. It includes mental disorders, infections and pathologies in modern nomenclature.

5. This repertory follows the Kent's grading of remedies.

6. More number of remedies. i.e., about 1800 remedies.

7. Rubrics like antibiotics, worse from; anesthesia, ailments from; artificial food aggravation; chemotherapy, side effects; hang-over; heroin, addiction from; etc. mentioned under the chapter Toxicity, are useful for day to day practice.

8. This repertory can be utilized for repertorizing all types of cases i.e. a case having prominent generals or particulars.

9. It is compact.

10. Chronologically arranged, so we find a rubric very easily and do not have to hunt.

11. It includes modern clinical and pathological conditions e.g.: Alzheimer's syndrome, polycystic ovaries, etc.

12. Word index is given for easy reference.

13. Inclusion of new remedies, nosodes, sarcodes and even bowel nosodes.

14. Ailments of Joints in general and individual joints, easy to refer as they are arranged as separate chapters.

15. Sections coming under each chapter are given at the chapter index itself.

- Lacks the superscript code references of the author who have contributed towards additions to Kent's repertory. Therefore it is very difficult to know the source of concerned data as well as remedy.

- There are some rubrics, which have been combined from the original Kent repertory. An example is combination of egotistical and Haughty into one rubric Egotistical haughty. The two words describe the characteristic, as originally perceived by Kent and belong to two separate rubrics.
- Sub rubric repeated. Page 186, URINATION, general, retarded, lying, can only pass urine while.
- Rubric alphabetically not arranged. Page 186, URINATION, general, retarded.

5. In abdomen epigastrium not represented well.

6. Main rubric not alphabetic, DELUSIONS, STEPPING

7. Same word different meaning. EARS, BORING, ABDOMEN, HARDNESS, COUGHING, SHARP

8. Reliability of new rubrics such as 'Aids'.

9. Misplacement of rubrics: eg. Axilla under Shoulder, Urethra under Bladder, Expectoration under Lungs.

10. Sub-rubrics coming under rubric 'Eruption' in different chapters are arranged in a scattered manner.

11. Even though many additions have been made, many omissions are also there. For example, Teeth, pain sound teeth in, is found in Kent but not in Murphy.

12. Many errors, technical as well as philosophical are there in this repertory. E.g.: Technical: A. Spelling mistakes and added letters.1. Female, discharge vaginal, girls, in little. Medicine Bufo is given as Bufo1.B. Other errors: Shoulders, pain, lying and its sub rubrics are given under Shoulder, Pain, lifting.

- Philosophical: mistakes in alphabetic arrangement.
- The third edition now contains 74 chapters, in 2,419 pages, 5.5 inches x 8.5 inches, on Bible paper in one volume.
- Over 20,000 new rubrics, and more than 100,000 new additions and updates, all in a small lightweight book for convenience.
- The third edition now contains 74 chapters, in 2,400 pages

New Chapters:

Cancer, Clinical, Fainting, Gall bladder, Speech, Spleen, Taste, Time, Vaccination, Weakness.

Deleted chapters:

Blood, Delusion, Diseases, Emergency, Environment, Nerves.

- This repertory can be used for all types of cases and any method can be followed to repertorise the case.
- Also it fits to the philosophy of general repertory with clinical approach.
- Also its abundance of rubrics especially in clinical, modern terminology along with provers symptom makes it more valuable.
- Only exception is its authenticity especially in latest clinical terms.

D. REPERTORIUM UNIVERSALE

Author: Dr. Roger Van Zandvoort

INTRODUCTION : C. von Bönninghausen's repertories, especially his Therapeutic Pocket Book have been used for more than 165 years by many masters of homeopathic practice. They have fallen into comparative disuse during the past 120 years because J.T. Kent and also C. Hering wrote strongly against them occasionally. Kent did so for economic reasons just to promote his own repertory and thus few homeopaths have knowledge of C. von Bönninghausen's philosophic background and practical principles of repertorization. The purpose is not to set forth the superiority of any one general repertory over another; but it is our desire to demonstrate the sound philosophy and practical application of C. von Bönninghausen's work to such states as the homeopath meets in everyday practice. Once its principles are assimilated and used and many times in combination with the more Kentian way of repertorizing.

A failure to grasp the concept and philosophical basis of what Hahnemann and Bönninghausen were seeking to achieve in the Therapeutic Pocketbook has most likely been the principal underlying reason for its falling into disuse. Some practitioners have mistaken their own lack of understanding for a failure in the work itself, and have gone on to compound the error by teaching this to others.

Over the past three decades much work has been carried out integrating and improving older and existing repertories, but the templates used to make these improvements are still largely based on the one created by Kent over a century ago. This has its limitations as the full potential of other methods of repertorisation, particularly Boenninghausen's can't be fully utilized in any single Repertory.

In 2002-3, the project took a new direction and a new structural arrangement of the repertory, the **Repertorium Universale** , was introduced. In this repertory, Kent's basic structure gave way to one which successfully married Kent's approach with that of the older sources. This allowed much fuller use to be made of methods such as Bönninghausen's and gave homeopaths far greater flexibility and versatility in the way they could approach the repertorisation of a case. The repertory allowed complete symptoms to be reliably constructed from the sum of their parts, rather than relying on finding an existing record of the exact, or closest possible symptom.

Boenninghausen technique has considerably greater flexibility and potential for solving cases that a repertory based only on complete recorded symptoms. This is because the complete symptom of the patient, whatever it might be, can be built from its components parts by the use of partial symptom rubrics, each of which is generally characteristic of remedy it contains. This is enormously useful in cases where very distinctive and characteristic symptoms can't be including in the repertorisation because it simply isn't in the repertory.

The *Repertorium Universale* differs from purely Kentian repertories. It still contains all the Kentian repertory information in its familiar form, but the alterations to its basic structure make it a far more flexible tool than one constrained to Kent's schema. The repertory is designed to work equally well with any number of different repertorisation strategies.

Boenninghausen's approach can be used as easily as Kent's, and it's ideally suited to the newer family/group-based thematic analytical techniques. This introduction and guide explains exactly how, where and why the *Repertorium Universale* differs from its predecessors and what benefits it offers which have been unavailable in any one single repertory until now.

PLAN AND CONSTRUCTION:

Most of Bönninghausen's published work is included in the comprehensive modern computerised "super-repertories" - the Complete Repertory and Synthesis. But their predominantly Kentian structure has made it difficult to use Bönninghausen's approach in conjunction with them. The problem of updating the more general rubrics with newer remedies (which aren't admitted directly to a rubric as a result of their provings) has been partially addressed in composite main rubrics (a feature of the Complete but not Synthesis), but this falls a long way short of a systematic updating of the entire repertory from the perspective of the "Bönninghausen Method."

This is the deficiency which Roger van Zandvoort is seeking to remedy in the Repertorium Universalis. What he has done with the structure of the repertory is essentially to turn the Kentian schema inside out. In Kent's schema, each major phenomenon is listed alphabetically within its appropriate main section with sub-rubrics qualifying sides, times, alternations, modifications (modalities, causations and concomitants), extensions and locations. Van Zandvoort has taken these qualifying dimensions and generalised them to section level as the first level of the hierarchy, followed by the phenomena according to the more familiar Kentian layout, so that the first level in each section now appears as blocks of qualifying dimensions, viz:

Alternating symptoms
1. Sides
2. Times
3. Modifications
4. Extending to
5. Location
6. Phenomena

The principal difference between the structure of Kent's Repertory and those compiled by Boenninghausen is in Kent's use of a defined hierarchy in the way he organises the indexing of the symptoms. All locations and modifications of symptoms (with the exception of some rubrics in the Generalities section) are dependent on a primary classification based on sensation. In other words, you can't find any location or modification unless it's describing a sensation, no matter how characteristic of a remedy that location or modification might be in its own right. Because of this, integration of Boenninghausen's rubrics which are independent of sensation (Locations, Sides, Times, Concomitants, Aggravations, Ameliorations, Alternations) can't be achieved in a Kentian-structured repertory, and it isn't possible to use Boenninghausen's technique with such a repertory.

In the **Repertorium Universale** nearly 1.5 million remedy additions have been made in over 180,000 rubrics with extensive cross-referencing. It includes all the features of the Complete Repertory . The grades of remedies — an indication of their reliability in the context of each symptom — have been re-classified and further clarified. The abbreviations of the remedy names have been corrected and synonyms reconciled. Most importantly, the re-structuring of the layout of rubrics makes it possible to use different repertorisation methods in a single search strategy. This makes the **Repertorium**

Universale a much more flexible tool for evaluating how closely a patient's symptoms match a given remedy's therapeutic profile in the Materia medica.

By re-structuring the format of the rubrics in the **Repertorium Universale** , both Kent's and Boenninghausen's models are accommodated and presented as a single fully integrated repertory. The Kentian-structured repertory (i.e. the Complete Repertory) has been nested within an expanded hierarchy which now includes Boenninghausen's rubrics in the primary classification of symptoms. This result in a repertory which effectively offers the best of both worlds — the greater precision of the complete symptoms found within the Kentian structure, plus the greater flexibility of symptom combination provided by the Boenninghausen-style rubrics.

Generalised partial rubrics have attracted a lot of criticism over the years, from Bönninghausen's day onwards, much of it resulting from an understanding which evidently misses the most important feature of these rubrics. All the remedies contained in these rubrics are there because that particular partial symptom has been found to be characteristic of the remedy in its own right, having been recorded as a feature of at least three separate and distinct symptoms produced or cured by the remedy. Using this criterion, all the Bönninghausen-style rubrics contained in the **Repertorium Universale** have been thoroughly and comprehensively updated with all the new remedies since his time.

SPECIAL FEATURES :

It is the largest Kentian style repertory. All remedies from sub rubrics represented in the main rubric and all remedies and rubric of the specific pains taken into the general pain rubric.

In the **Repertorium Universale** , the addition of all Boenninghausen's repertories has been completed, the Boenninghausen-specific rubrics have been updated with most if not all post-Boenninghausen material and the Kentian foundation finally gives way to a structure allowing an even balance between flexibility and precision.

Some exceptions to the updating process need mentioning. The Mind section contains two Boenninghausen rubrics which are added for completeness, but not updated. The first is Concomitant — remedies which feature mental alterations as a concomitant of physical symptoms. The second is General — remedies with a general affinity for the mental/emotional sphere. Updating will take place when (or if) Boenninghausen's criteria for inclusion are sourced. There is a similar Concomitant rubric in the Generalities section.

A further three sections have been introduced to the primary classification (Heart and Circulation, Blood, and Clinical) and the two Phenomena sections which were listed in their own right in editions of the Complete Repertory — Head Pain and Extremity Pain — have been reincorporated into the Head and Extremities sections. The separate section indexing Mirilli's themes, introduced in the Millennium edition of the Complete Repertory , is retained, now with more extensive cross-referencing and more remedies.

The "modalities" are impressively clear (Boenninghausen) while the repertory also offers a meaningful connection to the classical Kentian "phenomena". It is, in fact, a flexible tool, which enables him to adapt his clinical investigation to the phenomenological characteristics of a patient. That's why he consider Roger's work an actualization of a long-awaited, expanded approach to the patient, compatible with concepts of anthropological phenomenology.

Repertorium Universale also represents the "probabilistic" nature of any investigation of reality, as a consequence of the analogical relationship between the aspects we perceive of the universe. Every aspect investigated, has in fact, simultaneously, many different links and analogical connections to other parts and aspects. Every connected Modality, Alternating symptom, Side, Time, Extension to, and Location represents a virtual door to "Possible Worlds" (Patients/Remedies). Regardless of any common conceptual frames, limits and biases we may be bound by, **Repertorium Universale** offers an easy and clean structure to directly apply any repertorial search/approach."

Cross-references between rubrics have been thoroughly revised and increased, with the new repertory featuring more than double the number included in the last edition of the Complete Repertory .

Working with the Bönninghausen's approach also encourages a different perspective on the literature — patterns and themes are emphasized, which works well with the latest trends in analytical technique.

The grading system changes have been made to give a more accurate impression of the characteristic nature of symptoms recorded in proving — a frequent source of frustration for today's proving directors. Bönninghausen's criteria provide a clearer delineation between proving information (including herbal and toxicological data) and clinical confirmation. It gives a finer and more precise differentiation between the degrees and paves the way for further revisions in future editions of the repertory which will grade remedies according to even more precise criteria, removing all inconsistencies and confusion.

To make use of Boenninghausen's generalised rubrics, the symptoms of the case are constructed from the appropriate generalised partial symptom amongst the symptom modifications (Alternations, Sides, Times, Modalities, Extensions, Locations) plus Phenomena. These rubrics have been created for each section from Boenninghausen's original rubrics, including later additions from his handwritten works, and updated with all the newer remedies and clinical confirmations which qualify. They form the first level of the hierarchy in each section. Remedies only qualify for addition to these rubrics if the symptom quality is clearly characteristic of the remedy. This essential component — indeed guiding principle — of Boenninghausen's generalization process cannot be overemphasized, having been consistently overlooked by critics of the approach who rightly draw attention to instances where generalization is inappropriate. In the **Repertorium Universale** a symptom quality is regarded as characteristic if it appears in three or more separate symptoms, and has been added to the Boenninghausen-style rubrics on this basis, maintaining the highest degree found in any of its occurrences.

In the **Repertorium Universale** , it's now possible to use all methods within the one repertory, even to intermingle them in the one case if appropriate, or to use the generalised Boenninghausen-style rubrics to approach cases from a thematic angle (families, groups, etc). This effectively frees you to individualize the method to the case as precisely as you'd expect to individualize the remedy, drawing on a fully updated database of remedies.

E. PHOENIX REPERTORY

Author : Dr. J. P. S Bakshi

Phoenix:

A mythical bird with gorgeous plumage, fabled to be the only one of it's kind and to live five or six hundred years in the Arabian desert, after which it burnt itself to ashes on a funeral pyre ignited by the sun and fanned by it's own wings, rising from it's ashes with renewed youth to live through another cycle.

Dr. J. P. S Bakshi

- A renowned Homoeopathic physician. He has also specialized in Psychiatry.
- "Manual of Psychiatry" is his first publication.
- "The Phoenix Repertory", is his next publication in the year 1999. It was published by Cosmic Healers Pvt. Ltd, New Delhi in two volumes.

Major Sources

- S. Hahnemann
- Boenninghausen's Therapeutic pocket Book
- Boger's Boenninghausen's Characteristics and Repertory
- C.Hering, "The guiding symptoms of materia medica"
- Kent's Repertory
- Complete Repertory
- Synthetic Repertory
- Synthesis Repertory
- Kunzli's Repertory
- Sivaraman's Additions & Corrections to kent's Repertory

Plan and Construction

- Preface
- Contents
- Introduction
- Notes
- the Phoenix Repertory (Volume one/ two)
- Repertory Proper
- List of Remedies and Abbreviations
- List of Authors
- Notes

Repertory Proper

This Repertory follows Hahnemannian Anatomical schema. It can be classified as an " Alphabetical Systematic Repertory". Author has followed construction and philosophical background same as of Kent's Repertory with minor changes. The Repertory part is printed in two columns on each page.

Arrangement of remedies

- The number of remedies used in this Repertory are a total of 1600 remedies.
- Remedies are alphabetically arranged.
- Sources numbering in the form of a subscript following the remedy has been done:

E.g.; Coloc.1 (S. Hahnemann),

Calc.9 (Reference works),

Calc.54a(Knerr)

Grading of Remedies

Remedies have followed the four types of Typographies to indicate the grading of medicines:

- Remedies in plain type face are the first degree remedies

- Remedies in bold italics type face are the second degree remedies
- Remedies in BOLD UPPERCASE type face are the third degree remedies
- Remedies in BOLD UPPERCASE with underline type face are the fourth degree remedies

Arrangement of Rubrics

- There are a total of 1,25,514 rubrics.
- Rubrics are alphabetically arranged in the order of side, time, modality, extension and location.
- Main rubrics are given in CAPITAL BOLD.
- Sub rubrics are given in bold ordinary roman letters.
- Main and sub rubrics if continue to the next column, then they are mentioned above each column. Main rubrics in bold ordinary roman letters and sub rubrics in ordinary roman letters Symbols given after the rubric
- Rubric phrases taken from Kent's Repertory are marked with º (degree)
- Rubric phrases taken from Synthetic Repertory are marked with ~
- Different Cross references are separated with a small black dot
- And are closed in one bracket.
- Direct Cross references, where no remedies are mentioned, are marked with », thus referring to go to the mentioned rubric or rubrics.

Arrangement of Chapters

There are 38 Chapters. Every chapter starts from a new page and title of the chapter is mentioned in the center of the beginning of every chapter in Bold Title Uppercase. In the following pages, it is mentioned on the right upper corner of the right page, in ordinary Title Uppercase.

Volume one

There are 21 chapters:

- Mind
- Dreams
- Vertigo
- Head
- Eyes
- Vision
- Ears
- Hearing
- Nose
- Face
- Mouth
- Teeth
- External Throat
- Throat
- Larynx & Trachea
- Chest
- Respiration
- Cough
- Expectoration
- Stomach
- Abdomen

Volume two

There are 17 chapters:

- Rectum
- Stool
- Kidneys
- Bladder
- Urethra

- Urine
- Prostate
- Male
- Female
- Back
- Extremities
- Sleep
- Chill
- Fever
- Perspiration
- Skin
- Generalities

Mind Chapter

- There are 18,258 rubrics
- Latin and Greek terminology of fear are used:

  E. g., Acarophobia, Acrophobia, Ailurophobia, Algophobia, Cainotophobia, Claustrophobia, Gamophobia

- Rubrics not present in Kent: Ailments from; domination by others, a long history of:

  Ailments from; misfortune of others: Anger; vindictive Fear; AIDS, of

Special Features

- This repertory has 80,000 additions, 2 times the total number of rubrics in Kent and 4 times the number of mind rubrics than in Kent.
- The source of collected data is mentioned for each remedy, which makes the book reliable

- Many clinical rubrics are added to each chapter, it includes mental disorders, infections and pathologies in modern nomenclature
- This repertory can be utilized in repertorising all type of cases that is both with generals and particulars
- Repertory has followed the plan and construction of Kent's Repertory. Hence, it is easy to use this Repertory.

Criticism

- The Repertory contains many medicines. Majority of them are not well proved, though they have been added from authentic sources and there use cannot be definite and sure in clinical practice
- Some of the medicines are not available in common materia medica works, hence knowledge about these remedies remains incomplete
- Index for repertory is not given, which makes the rubric search difficult for beginners.

CONCLUSION

Creation of this Repertory has enriched our field, given it new vigour and vitality. As it is the latest repertory, it is worth to get a place on one's working table.

F. SYNTHETIC REPERTORY VOLUME I, II, III

Authors: Dr. med. Horst Barthel & Dr. med. Will Klunker

Horst Barthel constructed Volume I & II. Volume III is by Will Klunker (according to the front cover page)

Translator:

- German translation: Dr. Pierre Schmidt of Geneva
- French translation: Dr. med. Jacques Baur, Lyon with few additions.

Year of publication:

- 1ˢᵗ edition: 1973
- 2ⁿᵈ revised & improved edition: 1980 – 82
- 3 rd edition: 1987
- 4ᵗʰ improved edition reprint: 993

This repertory is published in **3 languages**: English, German and French

Number of remedies: 1594

1598 in the reprint edition, 1993 by B.Jain Publishers (P) ltd., New Delhi

Gradation of remedies

BOLD CAPITAL UNDERLINE

- 4 grades
- 1ˢᵗ grade:
- 2ⁿᵈ grade: **BOLD CAPITAL**
- 3ʳᵈ grade: **Small letter bold**
- 4ᵗʰ grade: small letter

Based mainly on (Author's index)

1) Kent. J.T
   - Kent's Repertory
   - Lectures on Homoeopathic Materia medica
   - New remedies
2) Knerr.C
   - Repertory of the Hering Guiding Symptoms of our Materia Medica
3) C.M.Boger
   - Boenninghausen's Characteristics and Repertory
   - Addition to kent's repertory
   - A synoptic key of the Materia Medica
4) Jahr G.H.R
   - Systematic Alphabetical Repertory of the Homoeopathic Remedy Doctrine
5) Gallavardin J.P
   - Psychisme et Homoeopathie
6) Stauffer.K
   - Symptom index
7) Schmidt.P
   - Annotations in Kent's repertory
   - Kent's Final General Repertory published by D.H.Chand.
   - His 50 years of clinical experience made him to introduce 4ᵗʰ grade to many drugs.
8) Boericke.O.E
   - Boericke's repertory
9) Stephenson.J
   - A Materia Medica and Repertory, Hahnemann's Provings 1924 – 1959
10) Mezger.J
   - Gesichetete Homeopathische Arznemittellehre – 35 reproven / new drugs

11) Allen.T.F
   - A general Symptom Register of the Homoeopathic Materia Medica

12) Clarke.J.H
   - A clinical Repertory of the Homoeopathic Materia Medica

13) The most recent drug provings published in the journals.

14) Julian.O.A
   - Matiere Medicale d' Homeotherapie of 1971
   - Dictionnaire de Materia Medicale de 130 Noveaux Homeotherapeutiques (2nd edition of the 1st book)

15) Kunzli.J – Supplements taken from the International Homoeopathic Literature.

16) Hahnemann.S
   - Materia Medica Pura
   - Chronic Diseases

This is the **first repertory** to use the numbering system to show the exact source of the sysmptoms or drugs. Numbering is done in superscript from after the drug.

No numbering for Kent's Repertory remedies.

- [1]mark for addition made in his own hand in Kent's repertory.
- [1'] for supplements from Kent's Lectures and New Remedies
- 2-14 respectively numbered as per the order of the author index.
- [1,5] or [1,7] Gallavardin's and Pierre Schmidt's experience made some drugz of Kent's repertory into higher grades.

- Asterisk sign '*' is used for symptoms refers to one of the 138 new collected rubrics of the index of Vol I and Vol II.

Philosophical background

Based on generals

The **first volume of synthetic repertory** deals with psychic symptoms:

Comparison of Kent Repertory with Synthetic at the level of mental generals
In Kent's repertory 528 mental rubrics are given where as in synthetic repertory 563 mental rubrics are given. Some new rubrics which are there in synthetic and are not there in Kent's

1.   ADULTEROUS
2.   ALERT
3.   AFFABILITY
4.   AGILITY, MENTAL
5.   AILMENTS FROM
6.   ANOREXIA MENTALIS
7.   BARGAINING
8.   BILIOUS DISPOSITION
9.   BUOYANCY
10. CORRUPT
11. COUNTRY DESIRE FOR
12. FINANCE APTITUDE FOR
13. PESSIMIST
14. POSTPONING
15. SELFLESSNESS
16. YIELDING DISPOSITION
17. UNRELIABLE
18. UNDIGNIFIED
19. TEARING
20. SUSCEPTIBILITY

Rubrics not present in Synthetic Repertory but present in Kent's repertory

1. ATTITUDE, assumes strange
2. BELLOWING
3. FRIGHT, complaints from
4. GROWLING like a dog
5. KNEELING and praying
6. MANIA A POTU
7. MIRTH, hilarity, liveliness, etc
8. NEW, objects seem
9. PIETY, nocturnal
10. POWER, love of
11. REPULSIVE mood
12. SEXUAL EXCESSES, mental symptoms from
13. SURPRISES, pleasant, affections after
14. UNFRIENDLY humour
15. UNOBSERVING
16. UNREAL
17. UNTRUTHFUL
18. WICKED disposition
19. WILD feeling in head

In addition to this lot of rubrics given with cross reference but some/no remedies in Kent were not present in Synthetic Repertory: 133 rubrics.

New remedies added to the old list given in Kent's repertory

1. Abrupt: Puls, Calc carb, Lyc, Sulph
2. Ailments from indignation: Ars
3. Anxiety in children: Cina
4. Egotism: Lyc, Verat
5. Fear of being alone: Asf, Nat carb
6. Fear of animals: Bell, Calc carb
7. Fear of his own shadow: Calc carb
8. Jealousy: Med
9. Desire to kill with knife: Lyc
10. Never laugh: Ars

Special features

- It consists only of general symptoms much more than Kent and thus helpful for Repertorisation where lot of general symptoms are present.
- Causative mental symptoms are brought together under one rubric called 'Ailments from' in Vol.1
- It consists of 1594 remedies and many more new rubrics than Kent.
- Sources from where the symptoms and drugs are taken are properly indicated by number.
- Huge reference: old, new, rare, and specific reference are possible.
- Helps in studying materia medica
- Published in 3 languages
- It represents synthesis of homoeopathic knowledge of the last 170 years
- Common errors like double entries, lack of clarity and wrong nomenclatures are corrected.
- Clinical rubrics are mentioned in various sections

Criticism

- Mental causative ailments are seperated but physical causative ailments are scattered in Vol II.
- This repertory is not useful for the cases which have complete particular symptoms.
- Though it's the enlarged version of Kent's repertory, in mind chapter 18 rubrics are missing.
- In a complete case we have to use 3 volume of Synthetic plus Kent's repertory for particulars and hence its not easy for a quick bed side reference.

G. PHATAK REPERTORY - A CONSICE REPERTORY OF HOMOEOPATHIC MEDICINES

Author : Dr.S.R.Phatak

This is an alphabetically arranged clinical type of repertory, covering the body as a whole. First edition of this repertory was published in 1963. The second enlarged and revised edition was published in 1977.The third is also called " revised enlarged edition" published in 2000. New additions of the rubrics are marked with ' + ' mark in the third edition.

Other important works of Dr. S.R. Phatak are:

- Repertory of biochemic remedies [English]
- Homoeopathic materia medica and repertory of homoeopathic medicines [Marathi]
- Materia medica of homoeopathic medicines [English]

Sources: the information is taken from authentic sources as well as from authors own experience, or by authorities like Dr Boger, Dr Kent, Dr Clark etc.

Plan & construction:

- In this repertory, the headings including mentals, generals, modalities, organs & their sub parts are all arranged in an alphabetical order. So first rubric is ABDOMEN affections in general. This is folllowed by sides,sensations eg :fist of a child moving as if; modalities,conditions eg: diabetes ,pneumonia,ascites etc.
- Causation is also mentioned here.eg: laparotomy after, pulmonary oedema after,operation for fistula
- Modalities & associated symptoms & cause of pains are given separately. eg: gripping, cramp,colic < arm raising

- Different character of pain is given under the sub rubric. Abdomen - pain- cutting Abdomen pain - gripping etc in alphabetical order.
- In the rubric ABDOMEN -EXTERNAL conditions of skin are given eg : cracks on skin.
- All the physiological & pathological conditions such as appetite,a version, desires, nausea, vomiting, thirst, fever,pulse etc are included in alphabetical order.eg : absent - minded,agarophobia etc.
- Cross-references are given wherever necessary.eg: all gone sensation-empty, bones brittle -see brittle
- In each rubric all important symptoms, their concomitants & modalities are given.
- For all general modalities & all particular modalities < & > are given.
- Boger created many general rubrics from some particular symptoms.All such rubrics are included in this work.eg: awkwardness
- The author has carried a few new headings from his experience eg:gait-unsteady
- In homoeopathy modalities & concomitants are most important factors for finding out a remedy.The author gathered all useful modalities from different standard repertories & are in included in this book.eg: holding breath >
- Grading according to their importance 1st →CAPITALS

2nd → italics

3rd → ordinary roman

- The modalities regarding position & posture of the patient is so much valuable. If the patient says that he feels better only when he assumes some strange position, this should be considered. This modality is not given in any of the standard repertories. This condition is given under attitude – bizarre ie, stange or unusual.

- Causation are given under < either general or particular.eg:anaemia – grief from.

Asthma-fright after

Cancer -smoke from.

- Appearance of symptoms one side or going up or downward - all these are given under the rubric - direction of symptom (86) here the sub rubrics like ascending, backward, diagonal, crosswise, here & there radiating etc.

- Appetite given as as a separate rubric under which many sub rubrics like capriciousness, easy satiety,increased hunger,vomitting on attempting to eat etc.

- Organs or parts of the body are mentioned as subrubrics & under which conditions occuring in these organs are mentioned with their cause & concomitants.

- The rubric AVERSION given as general aversion to various factors of life & aversion to various foods are given.

- Pathological & diagnostic terms are used as-bronchitis, malaria, measles, pneumonia.

- < & > by change of position is given as general rubric.

- Complaints of infants &children are given under the rubric CHILDREN & sub rubric as given alphabetically.

- Character of discharges are given in rubric discharges

- Medicines which antidote or remove the bad effects of narcotics are given under drug abuse of.The specific drug or corresponding antidote is given. Anaesthetic vapours-Acet.ac, Hep., Phos Anti- typhoid injections-Bapt Narcotics-Lache

Opium - Puls

- Sterility is found in female affections in general

- Gait is given as a rubric where different types of gait are mentioned.eg: dragging, limping, reeling, staggering etc.

- In dropsy due to different causes are given separately.

E.g.: dropsy alcoholism from dropsy heart affections with, kidney affections with,liver affections with.

- malposition of foetus with remedies for the different conditions caused by movements of foetus under the rubric- foetus.

MERITS : it is an alphabetical repertory- the headings including mentals,physical generals, modalities. Organs & their sub parts are all arranged according to their alphabetical order.

- In each rubric — location, sensation, modality & concomitants are given,also general modalities & mental symptoms. So we can use this for systematic repertorisation.

- Many rubrics especially modalities not found in other repertories are available here.

- The information is taken from authentic sources as well as from authors own experience. No drug is used unless the author has verified it in his own experience.
- The author has put forward a few new readings from his own experience. The rubric like blood pressure, bronchitis, bronchiectasis,colitis etc are very useful for nosological rubrics.
- Though this book is very small, it contains many rubrics which are not obtained in other books.

DEMERITS : there are limited numbers of rubrics as well as the remedies used in this concise repertory. Though graded, evaluation is not mentioned anywhere.

Important rubrics in Phatak's repertory:
1. Abdomen affections in
2. Abdomen external
3. Abortion
4. Abrupt
5. Abscess
6. Absent minded
7. Absent parts of body were
8. Absorbent action
9. Abusive, scolding
10. Aching (see under pain)
11. Acidity (see sour)
12. Acidosis
13. Acne (see eruptions)
14. Acromegaly
15. Actinomycosis
16. Active, agile
17. Activity fruitless
18. Acts, as if born tired
19. Acuminative, conical, growth, eruptions etc
20. Addision's disease
21. Adenoids
22. Adherent, internal sensation
23. Admonition agg
24. Adynamia (see weakness)
25. Aeroplane, flying in agg
26. Affectation
27. Affections, stipled
28. After pains
29. Agility (see active)
30. Agitation (see exitement)
31. Agony, anguish
32. Agoraphobia
33. Ague (see fever, intermittent)
34. Air blowing on part, through hole, as if
35. Air castles
36. Air hunger (see air open amel)
37. Air passages burning
38. Air - sickness (see Aeroplane flying agg)
39. Albuminous, glairy
40. Albuminuria
41. Alcoholic drinks agg
42. Alcoholism, acute
43. Alive sensation, as if
44. All - gone sensation (see empty)
45. Alone, when agg (see company amel)
46. Alternate days on agg (see day alternate agg)
47. Alternations mental
48. Alternation effects, states, sides, metastasis
49. Amaurosis (see vision paralysis of optic nerve)
50. Ambition, loss of (see indolence)

51. Amenorrhoea (see menses absent)
52. Ammoniacal odour (see discharges)
53. Amourous amative, erotic, lascivious
54. Anaemia
55. Analgesia (see numbness)
56. Anasarca (see dropsy)
57. Aneurism
58. Angel when well, devil when sick
59. Anger, vexation, irritability, fretfulness, bad temper
60. Angina pectoris
61. Angles (see skin, folds)
62. Animation (see cheerful)
63. Ankles
64. Annoyed easily
65. Anorexia (see appetite lost)
66. Answers aversion to (see aversion)
67. Antagonism with self
68. Anthrax
69. Anthropophobia, bashful (see shy)
70. Anticipations, and agg from
71. Anti social
72. Anus
73. Anxiety
74. Apathetic (see inactive)
75. Apathy (see indifference)
76. Aphasia (see speech lost)
77. Aphonia (see voice lost)
78. Apoplexy
79. Apparition (see vision fantastic)
80. Appendicitis (ileo - caecal region)
81. Appetite, affected in general
82. Arms (upper limbs)
83. Arrogance (see pride)
84. Arteriosclerosis
85. Arthralgia (see joints)

86. Arthritis deformans
87. Ascending agg
88. Ascites (see abdomen dropsy)
89. Asks for nothing
90. Asleep sensation
91. Asphyxia charcoal fumes from
92. Associated effects
93. Asthenopia (see under vision)
94. Asthma (bronchial)
95. Astigmatism (see under vision)
96. Athlete's foot
97. Atheroma (see calculi)
98. Athetosis
99. Atony
100. Atrophy
101. Attacks, recurrent (see relapses, recurrences)
102. Attention agg
103. Attitude, bizarre
104. Aura (see different sensation)
105. Automatic acts, motion
106. Autumn agg
107. Avaricious, greedy, miserly
108. Aversions, dislikes
109. Awakes, anger in
110. Awaking agg (mental symptoms)
111. Awkwardness (mental, physical)
112. Axillae
113. Back
114. Bad feel good and, by turns
115. Baldness (see head)
116. Ball lump knot etc
117. Band (see constriction)
118. Bandaged feeling
119. Barbers itch
120. Barking (like a dog)

121. Barometer

122. Bashful

123. Bathing aversion, to or from agg

124. Beads, like swelling

125. Bearing down (see pressing pain)

126. Beclouded (see comprehension difficult)

127. Beautiful things look

128. Bed, aversion, to

129. Bees stinging, as if

130. Behind, as if someone, or desire to look

131. Bending backwards, stretching limbs agg

132. Bereavement

133. Beriberi

134. Besides himself

135. Bewildered

136. Bilateral (see symmetrical)

137. Bile ducts

138. Bilharziasis

139. Bilious (see yellow)

140. Birth mark, naevi

141. Bite impulse to

142. Bites, cheeks or tongue

143. Biting chewing agg

144. Black dark (discharges, discolouration of skin, etc)

145. Black water fever

146. Bladder (urinary) affections in general

147. Blames himself

148. Bland (see discharges)

149. Bleeding agg

150. Blindness (see under vision)

151. Blisters (see eruptions vesicles)

152. Bloated (see puffiness)

153. Blondes

154. Blood boils

155. Blood pressure high

156. Blood sepsis (septic conditions, fever etc)

157. Blood vessels affections in general

158. Bloody (see discharges bloody)

159. Blowing nose agg

160. Blows, shocks, thrusts crash explosions, as from

161. Bluish, purple (discharges, discolouration of skin) etc

162. Board like sensation or feel

163. Boiling, as if

164. Boils

165. Boldness daring courageous

166. Bone affections, in general

167. Borrows troubles

168. Bounding internal (see alive sensation)

169. Bowels (see abdomen, and intestines)

170. Brain

171. Branny (see desquamation)

172. Breakfast agg

173. Breaking, broken (see pain things)

174. Breath cold

175. Breath again, cannot

176. Breathing deeply agg

177. Bregma

178. Briny (see salty, fishy)

179. Brittle, broken, feeling

180. Bronchiectasis, bronchorrhoea

181. Bronchitis

182. Brownish, rusty (discharges, discolouration of skin)

183. Brows

184. Bruised (see pain, sore)

185. Brunettes

186. Bubbles, sensation of
187. Bubo
188. Bullae
189. Bunions
190. Burning
191. Burns and scalds
192. Burnt
193. Burrowing, digging (see pain)
194. Bursae (see pain)
195. Business failure
196. Busy, when (see occupation) amel
197. Buttocks
198. Buzzing (see humming)
199. Calculi (urinary, biliary etc)
200. Calf
201. Callosities
202. Cancer
203. Canthi (eyes of)
204. Cap sensation
205. Capricious (see changing moods and appetite)
206. Carbuncle
207. Care and worry
208. Caresses agg
209. Caries (see under bones)
210. Carphology (picking at bed clothes, nervous picking)
211. Carried, wants to be
212. Caries things, from one place to another and back again
213. Carrying burdens agg
214. Car sickness
215. Cartilage
216. Caruncle see urethra)
217. Catalepsy
218. Cataract (see lens)
219. Catheterism
220. Caution
221. Celibacy
222. Cellars, vaulted places
223. Cellular tissue (cellulitis, etc)
224. Censorious
225. Cephalhaematoma
226. Cerobro - spinal axis
227. Cervix (uterus) cancer
228. Chagrin (see mortification)
229. Chancre hard
230. Change of position agg
231. Changing moods, erratic
232. Chaps (see cracks)
233. Charcoal fumes, ill effects
234. Cheeks
235. Cheerful
236. Cheesy, odour
237. Chest and lungs
238. Chewing
239. Chicken pox
240. Chilblains
241. Child bed
242. Childish, foolish
243. Children infants
244. Chill
245. Chilled from exposure to cold agg
246. Chin
247. Chloasmae
248. Chloroform agg
249. Choking (see throat)
250. Cholera
251. Chordee
252. Chorea
253. Choroid

254. Chronicity
255. Cicatrices
256. Circulation (see blood)
257. Clairvoyance
258. Claustrophobia (see fear narrow places)
259. Clavicle
260. Clavus (see plug)
261. Climaxis
262. Clitoris
263. Clothes cold
264. Cloudy weather agg
265. Clutching sensation
266. Coal gas agg
267. Coat, wears in summer, hot weather
268. Coated or furred as if
269. Cobweb sensation
270. Coccyx
271. Coition, aversion to (males)
272. Cold agg
273. Coldness
274. Colds (see coryza)
275. Colic (see pain, cramping and flatulence)
276. Colitis mucosa
277. Collapse (rapid, prostration)
278. Collar (see pressure of clothes around neck) agg
279. Colliquative states
280. Colours bright agg
281. Coma (see unconsiousness)
282. Come and go (see pain, fleeting)
283. Company crowd agg
284. Complaining, lamenting
285. Complaints, describe, cannot properly
286. Complexion clears
287. Compression
288. Concentration, difficult
289. Concussions
290. Condiments (see food)
291. Condyles (see under bones)
292. Condylomata (see fungus growth)
293. Confidence, want of self
294. Confusion, incoherence muddled
295. Congestion
296. Conical formation
297. Conjunctiva
298. Conscience, terror of
299. Consolation agg
300. Conspiracies. Suspects against him, there were
301. Constipation agg
302. Constipation (remedies in general)
303. Constriction, band, gathered together etc
304. Consumption, tuberculosis
305. Contempt, holds every thing in
306. Contemptuous scornful
307. Continence agg
308. Contortion, distortions
309. Contraction
310. Contractures (see strictures)
311. Contradict, disposition, to
312. Contradictions, intolerant of agg
313. Contradictory and alternating states
314. Contrariness
315. Control lacks
316. Conversation agg
317. Convulsions, spasms
318. Co-ordination disturbed
319. Copper colour (discharge, skin, etc)
320. Cornea, affections, in general
321. Corns (see callosities)
322. Corpulence (see obesity)

323. Corroding (see discharges acrid)

324. Coryza

325. Cottony feeling

326. Cough, remedies in general

327. Coughing agg

328. Counts continuously

329. Courageous (see boldness)

330. Covers agg (see also heat agg) cold application, amel

331. Cowardly (see anthropophobia)

332. Cracking joints in (see joints)

333. Crackling like tinsel

334. Cracks, fissures, chaps (see also skin)

335. Crafty (see deceitful)

336. Cramp (see pain crampy)

337. Crash (see blows)

338. Craving (see also desires)

339. Crazy (see insanity)

340. Creeping, running as of a mouse, etc

341. Crepitation

342. Cretinism

343. Cries, shrieks, screams (see also weeps, sorrows)

344. Crime committed, as if

345. Critical, exacting

346. Criticise, every thing wants to

347. Crossing limbs agg

348. Crossness (see anger)

349. Croup

350. Crowd (see company)

351. Cruelty

352. Crushing

353. Crusta lactea

354. Crusts, scabs

355. Cunning (see deceitful)

356. Cupped

357. Curdy (see discharges)

358. Cursing

359. Curvature (see bones, spine)

360. Cutting (see under pain)

361. Cyanosis (see bluish)

362. Cynical

363. Cystitis (see bladder inflamed)

364. Cysts

365. Damp, cold agg

366. Dampness, wet weather

367. Dancing

368. Dandruff

369. Dark (see black)

370. Darkness agg

371. Darting (see pain, darting)

372. Day alternate on agg

373. Day blindness

374. Dazed (see bilwildered, dull)

375. Dead look

376. Deadness

377. Dead thinks, he is

378. Deafness (see hearing)

379. Death agony

380. Debauchery

381. Debility (see weakness)

382. Deceitful, tricky, duplicity

383. Deceived, always being

384. Decomposition

385. Decubitus (see bed sores)

386. Deeds he could do great

387. Defined

388. Degeneration

389. Dejected (see despair, sadness and sorrow)

390. Delicate, tender, sickly

391. Delirium

392. Deltoid
393. Delusions (see imaginations, perception changed)
394. Dementia
395. Dentition
396. Depravity (see moral perversion)
397. Depression (see sadness)
398. Dermatalgia (see skin painful)
399. Dermoid
400. Descending agg
401. Desires (see also craving)
402. Despair hopelessness
403. Desquamation, branny, sclay etc
404. Desperate
405. Despondent
406. Destructive
407. Determined
408. Development
409. Diabetes, insipidus (see urine profuse)
410. Diaphragm
411. Diarrhoea
412. Digestion, affected
413. Digging (see pain, boring)
414. Dinner agg
415. Diplopia (see vision, double)
416. Dipsomania (see delirium tremens)
417. Diphtheria
418. Direction of symptoms
419. Dirty (see gray)
420. Disappointment
421. Disbehaviour of others (see misdeeds)
422. Discharges, loss of vital fluids agg
423. Discoloured (see under different colours, and mottled)
424. Discontent
425. Discordant (see confusion, co-ordination disturbed)
426. Discouraged (see despair)
427. Disgust (see aversion)
428. Dislocated, sprained as if
429. Dislocation easy, spontaneous
430. Disobedience
431. Disorderly
432. Displeased (see discontent)
433. Displeasure, reserved (see under reserved)
434. Dissatisfied (see discontent)
435. Distension, feeling of (see swelled, enlarged as if)
436. Distortions (see contortions)
437. Distraction, cannot collect ideas, concentration difficult
438. Distrustful (see suspicious)
439. Diversion amel
440. Domineering
441. Dotage
442. Doubting people
443. Downward (see under directions)
444. Draft agg (see wind agg)
445. Dragging, sensation
446. Drawing (see pain drawing)
447. Drawn back (see retraction)
448. Dreaminess, reverie, ecstasy
449. Dreams
450. Dreamy (see dreaminess)
451. Drinking agg
452. Drinks cold agg and amel (see under food)
453. Driving (see riding)
454. Dropping like water (see trickling)
455. Drops things (see awkward)
456. Dropsy edema

457. Drowsiness (see sleepiness)
458. Drugs, abuse of in general
459. Drunkards
460. Dry clear or cold weather agg
461. Dryness
462. Duality, in places, separated as if someone else
463. Dull, beclouded, difficult comprehension, stupified
464. Duodenum, affections of
465. Duplicity (see deceitful)
466. Dusk (see twilight)
467. Dusky colour (pale)
468. Dust, feather, as of
469. Dwarfish
470. Dysentery
471. Dysmenorrhoea (see menses painful)
472. Dyspepsia (see digestion affected)
473. Dyspepsia (see digestion affected)
474. Dysphagia (see swallowing difficult)
475. Dyspnoea (see respiration difficult and asthma)
476. Dysruia (see urination, difficult)
477. Ears
478. Eat, aversion, or refusal to
479. Eating agg
480. Ebullitions (see waves)
481. Ecchymosis, petechiae
482. Eclampsia
483. Ecstasy (dreaminess)
484. Ectropion (eyelids turned up)
485. Eczema
486. Edge, on, as if
487. Effects, single (see single parts)
488. Effusion, deposit
489. Egg albumin dried on, as if
490. Egoism (see pompous)
491. Elbows
492. Electric shock agg
493. Electricity amel
494. Elephantiasis
495. Elevating, limbs amel (see also hanging down limbs agg)
496. Elongated, as if
497. Emaciation, atrophy
498. Embarrassment agg
499. Embraces
500. Embolism
501. Emission al (see seminal emission)
502. Emotion
503. Emotions, mental excitement agg
504. Emphysema (see chest)
505. Empty, hollow, sinking
506. Emprosthotonus
507. Empyema (see under chest)
508. Empyocele
509. Enamel thin
510. Enervated (see delicate)
511. Enlarged, swelled, as if
512. Entropion (eyelids turned down)
513. Enuresis (see urination involuntary, and bed wetting)
514. Envy (see jealousy)
515. Epigastrium
516. Epilepsy (see convulsions)
517. Epithelioma (see cancer)
518. Epulis
519. Erection (of penis)
520. Erethism false
521. Erotic (see amorous)
522. Erratic (see changing moods)
523. Errors, diet, in agg

524. Eructation

525. Eruptions (tendency to)

526. Erysipelas

527. Erythema (see under eruptions)

528. Escape, impulse to

529. Eustachian tubes

530. Exacting (see critical)

531. Exaggerates, her symptoms

532. Exaltation (see cheerful)

533. Exanthemata, in general

534. Excessive use (see overuse)

535. Excitable (see anger)

536. Excitement mental, nervous

537. Excoriation (see discharges acrid)

538. Excrescences (fungus growth)

539. Excretions (see discharges)

540. Exertion mental agg

541. Exhalation agg

542. Exhaustion (see weakness)

543. Exhilaration (see cheerful)

544. Exostosis (see bones)

545. Exopthalmic goitre (see goitre)

546. Expectoration (see discharges)

547. Expiration (see exhalation)

548. Explosions (see blows and shattered)

549. Express herself, cannot

550. Expression (see face)

551. Extension (see stretching)

552. Extreme goes, to

553. Extremities (see arms)

554. Exudation (see effusion)

555. Eyebrows (see brows)

556. Eyelids

557. Eyes

558. Face

559. Fag, enervation (see delicate)

560. Failure, feels himself a

561. Faint, fainting (see also unconscious)

562. Falling

563. Faltering (see hesitates)

564. Fallopian tubes, inflammation of (salpingitis)

565. Fanaticism

566. Fancies (see perceptions changed)

567. Fanned, as if (see air, blowing, on part)

568. Fanning agg

569. Fantasy (see imaginations)

570. Far off feeling

571. Fastidious

572. Fasting agg

573. Fatigue agg

574. Fats (see food)

575. Fatty (see greasy)

576. Fauces, itching

577. Fault finding

578. Favus (see under eruptions)

579. Fear, anxiety, fright

580. Fearlessness (see boldness)

581. Feather (see dust)

582. Feather bed agg

583. Feeble (see weak)

584. Feels too hot (see heat agg)

585. Feet

586. Feigning sick (see malingering)

587. Felon (see fingers)

588. Females affections in general

589. Female organs in general

590. Ferocious (see delirium, maniacal)

591. Festering, as if

592. Festination

593. Fever

594. Fibroid tissue, ligaments

595. Fickle (see persevere cannot)

596. Fidgety

597. Figwarts (see fungus growths)

598. Film (see valve)

599. Financial loss agg

600. Fine pain (see pain stitching, needles, hair, hair sensation, thread sensation)

601. Fingers

602. Firelike (see burning fiery)

603. Fishy odour, taste etc

604. Fissure (see cracks)

605. Fistula

606. Fitful (see changing moods)

607. Fit of passion

608. Fixed ideas (see ideas)

609. Flabby feeling (see relaxation)

610. Flatulence

611. Flatus back, felt, in

612. Fleeting pains (see under pain)

613. Fleshy (see new growths, fungus growths)

614. Flexures (see skin, folds)

615. Floating, flying as if

616. Flowing (see tricking as of water)

617. Fluctuation (see waves)

618. Fluidity (see discharges)

619. Flushes (see waves)

620. Fluttering (see vibrations)

621. Flying to pieces (see shattered)

622. Foamy, frothy (see discharges foamy)

623. Foetid (see offensive)

624. Foetus, expels, dead

625. Fogs (see cloudy weather)

626. Folds (see skin)

627. Fontanalles (see under children)

628. Food and drinks agg and amel

629. Foolish (see childish, silly)

630. Forced apart (see separated as if)

631. Forceps delivery after

632. Fore arm (see under arms)

633. Foreboding (see fear of future)

634. Fore head

635. Foreign bodies

636. Forgetful (see memory bad)

637. Forgets errand

638. Forgotten something, constantly as if, he had

639. Formication crawling (see also skin)

640. Forsaken, lonely

641. Fractures (see bones broken, brittle)

642. Fragile (see broken feeling and bones brittle)

643. Frail as if body were

644. Frantic (see besides himself)

645. Freckles (see under eruptions)

646. Fretful (see anger)

647. Friction agg

648. Fright (see fear, emotions agg)

649. Frightened easily

650. Frost air agg

651. Frothy (see discharges foamy)

652. Fullness (see congestion)

653. Fumes (see vapour)

654. Fungus growth, Excrescences, warts, condylomata

655. Furibund (see delirium maniacal)

656. Furry (see coated)

657. Fury (see rage)

658. Fussy

659. Gagging

660. Gait, body trembles while walking

661. Gall bladder burning

662. Ganglia bursae
663. Gangrene
664. Gargling agg
665. Garlicky, odour of discharges, taste, etc
666. Gastric fever (see fever)
667. Gastritis
668. Gathered together (see constriction)
669. Gay (see cheerful)
670. Gelatinous (see discharges)
671. Genitals (in general, both sexes)
672. Gentle (see timid)
673. Gestures, makes
674. Ghosts (see fear)
675. Giddy (see vertigo)
676. Girdle pains (see under pain)
677. Girls (see puberty)
678. Glabella, aching, fullness and
679. Glands (in general)
680. Glans (penis)
681. Glaucoma (see under eye)
682. Gleet (see urethra, discharge gleety)
683. Glistening, shining
684. Globus (see ball, hysteria)
685. Gloomy (see sad)
686. Glossitis (see inflammation, tongue)
687. Glottis spasms of (laryngismus stridulus)
688. Gluey (see discharges gluey)
689. Gluttony
690. Gnawing (see pain gnawing)
691. Godless, want of religious feeling (see irreligious)
692. Goitre
693. Gonorrhoea
694. Goose skin
695. Gossiping
696. Gout
697. Gracile
698. Granular appearance
699. Granulation poor
700. Grapes like (see growth)
701. Grasped and relaxed (see opening and shutting)
702. Grasping agg (see fingers working with)
703. Gray, dirty (discharges, discolouration etc)
704. Greasy, oily, fatty (skin discharges etc)
705. Greedy (see avaricious)
706. Green, greenish (skin discharges etc)
707. Grief sorrow
708. Grimaces
709. Grinding (see pain cramping)
710. Gristly
711. Grit want of
712. Gritty feeling
713. Groaning (see moaning)
714. Groins
715. Groping in dark, as if
716. Ground gives way
717. Growing pains
718. Growling (see howling)
719. Growth, affected, disorders of
720. Growths new, tumours etc (see cancer, cysts)
721. Grumbling
722. Guilt, sense of
723. Gullet (see esophagus)
724. Gummata
725. Gummy (see discharges, gluey)
726. Gums
727. Gurgling

728. Gushing
729. Habits, intemperate agg
730. Hacking, like a hatchet
731. Haematemesis (see vomiting, blood, and haemorrhage)
732. Haematocele
733. Haematodes
734. Haematoma
735. Haematuria
736. Haemophilia
737. Haemoptysis (see haemorrhage)
738. Haemorrhage (see bloody discharges)
739. Haemorrhoids (see piles)
740. Hair affections of
741. Hair combing of brushing agg
742. Hallucinations (see perceptions changed and imaginations
743. Hammering (see pain, hammering, head)
744. Hamstrings, short, tense
745. Hand laying on part amel
746. Hands
747. Hanging affected parts agg and amel (see hanging limbs agg and amel)
748. Happy seeing ohters agg
749. Hard bed sensation (see bed pain, see pain aching)
750. Hardness, induration
751. Harsh
752. Haste (see hurry)
753. Hateful
754. Hatred (see malice)
755. Haughty (see insolent)
756. Hauteur (see pride)
757. Hawking (mucus)
758. Hay fever (see coryza annual)

759. Head affections in general
760. Head external (scalp and skull)
761. Head strong (see stubborn)
762. Healing difficult (wounds, ulcers, etc)
763. Hearing acute, sensitive to noise
764. Hearing talk agg (see talk hearing agg)
765. Heart
766. Heart burn
767. Heat agg (feels too hot)
768. Heat (see burning, fever)
769. Heated by fire, sun
770. Heaviness, load
771. Held being amel (see holding amel)
772. Hemicrania (see head, one sided symptoms)
773. Hemiopia (see vision half)
774. Hemiplegia (see also paralysis)
775. Here and there (see directions)
776. Hernia
777. Hiccough
778. Hide desire to
779. High living
780. Hip-joint
781. Hives (see urticaria)
782. Hoarseness (see voice)
783. Hodgkin's disease
784. Holding or being held amel
785. Hole, blowing through (see air blowing through)
786. Hollow (see empty)
787. Homesick
788. Honour wounded
789. Hook worm disease
790. Hopeful
791. Hopeless (see despair)
792. Horny (see growth, eruptions)

793. Horripilation (see goose skin)

794. Horror

795. Horse back (see riding on horse back)

796. Hot application amel

797. Hour exact agg (see periodicity)

798. House in agg

799. Howling

800. Humerus aching, right

801. Humid damp weather agg

802. Humming, buzzing, whizzing

803. Hunger (see appetite)

804. Hurry, impatience

805. Hurt, fears being

806. Hydrarthrosis (see water in joints)

807. Hydrocele

808. Hydrocephalus

809. Hydrogenoid

810. Hypochondriasis

811. Hypocrisy

812. Hypogastrium

813. Hypostasis

814. Hysteria

815. Icthyosis

816. Ice factory complaints

817. Icy cold (see coldness, icy)

818. Ideas (see imaginations)

It is difficult for a homeopath to remember all the huge works of the masters.

- To solve this problem masters have prepared books with specific symptoms related to a remedy in few key points –Repertory.

- But this is not the final solution for selection of similimum. Because to do Repertorization manually it takes many hours.

- It was at this time that many pioneers started to contemplate on idea of putting most commonly used generals symptoms and particular symptoms on a piece of paper- Card Repertories

- Computer technology has totally changed the way of thinking the field of Alternative Medicine like Homeopathy, it has taken computers into its fold.

- In homoeopathy, which is benefited most is the repertory, by working out a case in shortest time and arriving at the similimum is at the fingertip.

- In the year 1982, some Homeopaths from USA and Britain had tried to solve this problem by using computers in homeopathic repertorization and for the first time they designed computer program.

- With the help of computer program homeopaths are now able to get each line of the required information in both Repertories and Materia Medica.

- After emergence of software there are different software available to the Profession and each one has got its unique features.

- Like repertories computers are also gives the information what we feed, so one must have thorough knowledge, study in depth, and acquaintance with the software for doing Repertorization and to utilize them properly.

- So we need to know what are the mechanical aided repertories available to the profession. The details about those software's will help us to choose the right one.

A. AUTOVISUAL REPERTORY

In this type mechanical assistance is required to use various repertories.

- Auto visual miasmatic repertory
- Auto visual homoeopathic repertory
- Though the name of the book repertory has been given, but actually it is a device of repertorization, formulated by Dr. Ramanlal P. Patel of Kollyan, Kerala, India.
- Auto visual homoeopathic repertory is mechanized computer developed by Dr. Ramanlal P. Patel in 1972. Auto visual repertory is more cheap, simple, and most reliable than present day complex computer.

CONSTRUCTION OF AUTO VISUAL REPERTORY

This repertory has two main components:
1) Auto strip.
2) Auto visual apparatus.

AUTO STRIP

- In this repertory there are 5505 auto strips.Each auto strip has a number 1,2,3,4 on the top representing rubrics based on Kent's repertory. In many places auto strips are marked A, B, C along with numbers like, 70a, 104b, 131b etc. these are new additions in Kent's repertory.auto strips are grooved at several places. Each groove on the auto strip represents corresponding homoeopathic medicines in apparatus. Grooves are different colors indicating grading of medicines. E.g. BOLD CAPITAL- red

colored, italics- yellow color, roman- black color. These grades are compared with BTPB grading.

- Besides this there are 2 heavy grooves (green) one at the top and one at the bottom of the auto strip as guidelines to match with the guidelines of auto visual apparatus. Also by different colures of number symptoms are graded as Generals- Red colored, Particulars- Black colored, which help for selection of symptoms for Repertorization.

AUTO VISUAL APPARATUS

- This apparatus is based on Hahnemann's original hand written repertory. Where all symptoms must be written in such a way that one can separate every one of them by cutting them up and pasting them in alphabetical order for the purpose of printings.
- Auto visual apparatus is something just like idea of Haemoglobinometer, where the percentage is counted by matching the lines of scale with measuring test -tube.

Dr. Patel has prepared the 3rd apparatus it's nothing but the hand book of repertory which contain their rubric with their code numbers, arranged in systemic manner with an index. For easy reference in both cases the page numbers of Kent's repertory are given along side.

This apparatus has 435 medicines on it in numerical order from above downwards. Each medicine is provided with code number. This apparatus is constructed in such a way that just likes arrangement of auto strips. The strips are put in to a reading device, which stakes them allowing the lines to be seen clearly. Lines are which common to majority auto strips originated from code number of medicines, are considered as group of indicated remedies for given case.

This group is considering for final differentiation with Materia Medica. The wooden box, filled with the 5505 plastic strips, is about 2 feet square and 7 inches deep, made from a very dense native Indian wood; it weighs close to 90 pounds.

WORKING

- After case taking, evaluations and eliminations of the unimportant symptoms

- Refer the selected symptoms as rubrics in the handbook of Auto visual homoeopathic repertory with their code numbers auto strips numbers representing the selected rubrics are taken out from the auto strip box.

- Arrange the rubrics numbers in the order of importance.

B. HOMOEOPATHIC CALCULATOR TECHNIQUE

- This is actually not a machine. It is a simple book working like a calculator and it contains two parts:
  1) The Rubric part.
  2) The Calculator part.
- Rubric part contains the rubrics with their code Nos arranged in a definite process, so that hunting the rubrics and their code numbers become easy.
- Calculator part contains the names of the medicines as headings of the chapter, which are subdivided into several sub chapters according to the calculator.
- After evaluating the rubrics, record the rubrics one below the other with their code Nos given in the book.
- Now read the rubrics again and again and arrive at 8- 10 remedies with the knowledge of Materia Medica or select one very strong rubric without which prescribing is impossible, open the repertory and note the remedies in it (if many remedies are there discard the lower grades) or select 2 or 3 very important rubrics use the thumb and finger method and record the remedies.

- Now, the rubrics with code numbers are ready and the expected result medicines also are ready. Now open the page of the selected remedy in the handbook and record the grades against the rubric code number. Now you have a small tabulation form. Now add up all the total matching and total grades of each remedy.

Dr. D. Tarafder has prepared 3 full pledged calculator

1) Calculator from Sankaran's pocket repertory,
2) Calculator from BTPB
3) Calculator from Kent's repertory.

C. COIN PLAYING REPERTORY

Author: Dr. D. Tarafdar

- It is economic, time saving enjoyable play and work for finding out the correct prescription by Arithmetic calculation. By this process one can repertorise as many cases as he likes by a single set.

- It consists of
  1. Card Board
  2. Coin

1. On the card board, different medicines are written in the respective columns on the corner of the board.

2. The coins are in four colors, Red for 5 and 3 marks, blue for 4 and 2 marks, Green for 3 and 1 marks and black for 2 marks.

3. Technique –
   1. Take a small piece of paper on which note down the rubrics and their pg no. of the Repertory book that you will use.
   2. Read the rubrics and the medicines and place the coins in the specified rooms.
   3. Lastly look for highest peaks and identify them.
   4. Count the number of coins in highest peaks, total matchings and count their total values.
   5. Analyze or go to MM. Enjoy repertory as a game to play.

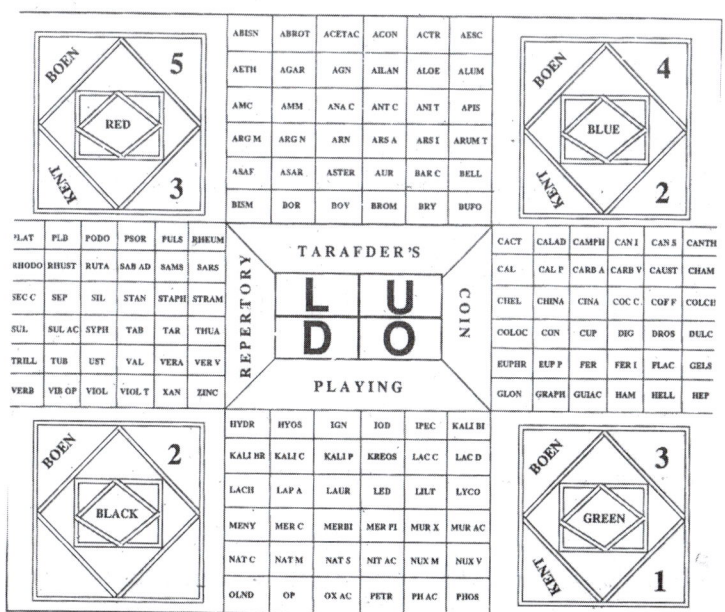

D. COMPUTER REPERTORIES

I. MAC REPERTORY

Synergy's repertorization tool, **Mac Repertory**, makes it easy to quickly select and analyze rubrics, get ideas for remedies, check the materia medica, do some research and feel confident about your prescriptions.

MacRepertory combines a solid, traditional approach to repertorization with dozens of inspirational features. Advanced analysis tools feature family graphs at your fingertips; keyword and remedy searches with features like the Theme Palette combine the best of Boenninghausen's generalism with Kent's specificity, with remedy comparison by family as well as single remedy. You'll immediately find you are prescribing more accurately.

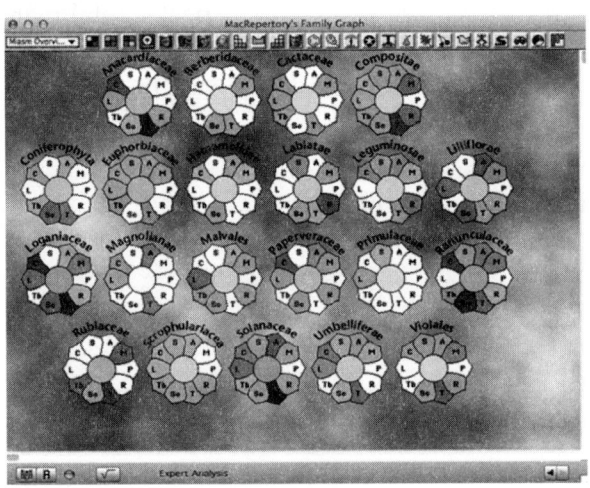

FEATURES

Mac & Windows Compatibility

Full compatibility with Mac OSX 10.6/10.7/10.8/10.9 and Windows 7 and 8. Now fully downloadable via Internet.

Friendly

User friendly and easy to use.

Collecting Rubrics

Collect your symptoms with a click; organize groups of symptoms into themes.

Analyzing

Analyze your case through clear graphs and multiple strategies.

Creating Graphs

Use graph limits to show predefined families and groups.

Comparing Concepts

Differentiate between remedies, groups and families using hundreds of concepts.

Communicate

Communicate with Reference Works program to improve your case analysis.

Family Dynamics

Use over 100 family graphs to look at your cases from many perspectives.

Do It Your Way

Design your own strategies, graphs, families and colours and make your own additions and changes to the repertories and personal keynotes.

Crossing Rubrics

Cross your cases' rubrics in the Elimination Tool to illuminate the remedies that run through your cases.

Case Management

Save your cases to the patient charts interface for future follow-up.

Materia Medica

Verify your remedies in the materia medica library of old and modern masters.

Discover Families

Follow and use masters' research in order to solve your cases and study families.

Research

Do research like the Masters. Conduct advanced and sophisticated searches of remedies & words in the repertory and study the nature of the remedies through their symptoms.

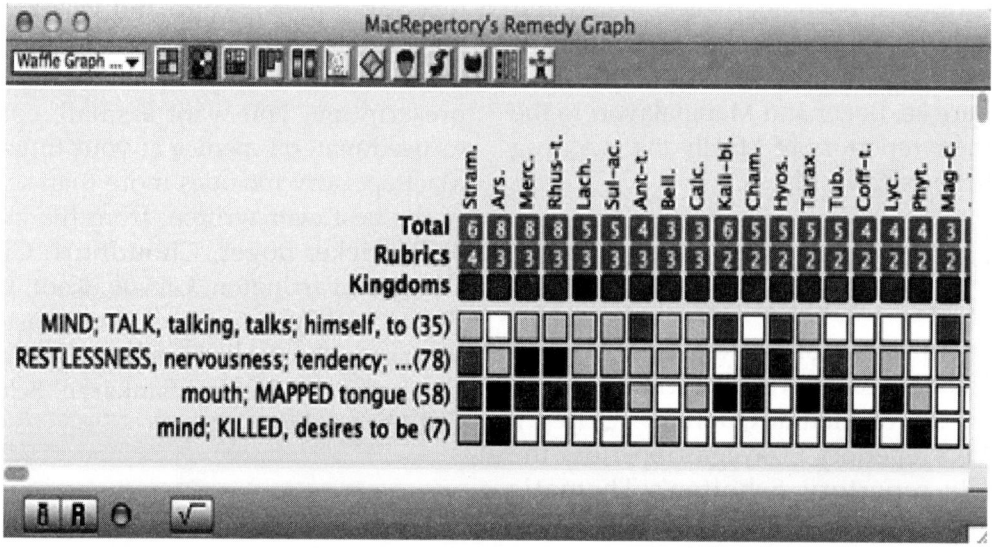

MAC REPERTORY LIBRARY

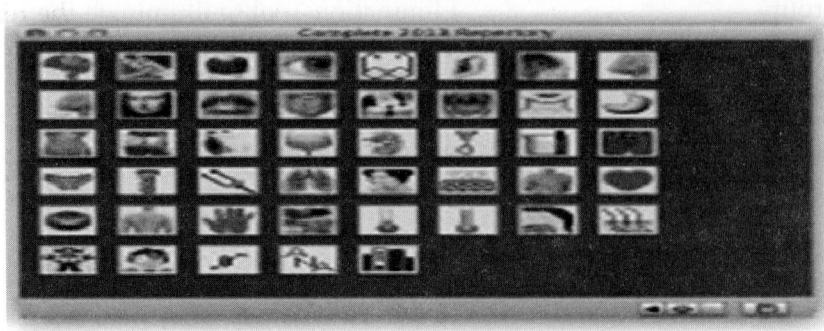

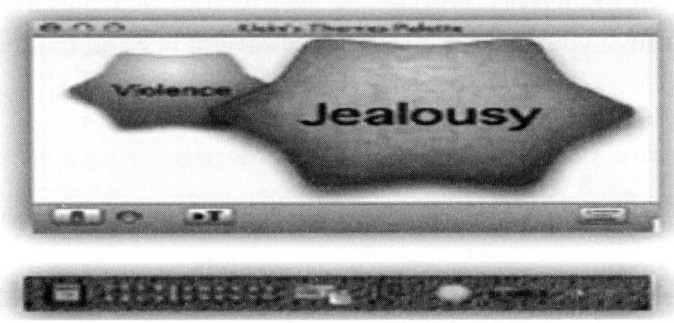

With more than 35 repertories, MacRepertory covers every aspect of homeopathy: from the general classic repertories of Boenninghausen, Allen and Kent to the focused classics of Knerr, Jahr and Boericke. From the essential repertories of Boericke, Boger and Mangialavori to the thematic repertory of Mirilli and the drug side-effects from Marsh.

Of course, we also have the world's most comprehensive repertory, Zandvoort's Complete, in its different forms.

In the Full library of MacRepertory, you can find modern repertories like Jeremy Sherr's Repertory of Mental Qualities (Q Rep.), Phatak's repertory, Eizayaga's repertory, the Family repertory, Scholten's Thematic repertory, Murphy's repertory (3rd Ed),

specific repertories for thyroid problems, AIDS, diabetes and sexual dysfunction and even Bach Flower and dream proving repertories plus Pitcairn and Jensen's New World Veterinary repertory! At the point that you're ready to confirm your prescription, you want a small, concise, focused materia medica at your fingertips. MacRepertory includes more than seventy of the best ever written: from the classics of Boericke, Boger, Choudhuri, Clarke, Dunham, Farrington, Gibson, Kent, Lippe, Phatak and Tyler to the modern masters of Morrison (both the Desktop Guide and Companion), Murphy, Sankaran, Scholten and Vermeulen.

II. HOMPATH CLASSIC

The Hompath Classic ver 8.0 is a Premium Collection of 11 modules, which effectively help the Homeopathic Practitioner to use it as his Intelligent Assistant to analyze their cases and arrive at the Correct Similimum thereby getting faster results and increasing their practice.

The unique benefits that a Practitioner gets when using the Premium Collection are outlined briefly below.

1. Educate patients in their own language and save time repeating instructions. This reduces hassles of repeating instructions to patients by printing Patient Instructions from over 200 Patient Instructions.

2. Reduces your prescription time by Instant Repertorisation. You need to enter the symptom the way the patient narrates them and you get the repertorisation table at the same time. This unique benefit is offered by the "Quik Reperotrisation" feature in Classic version 8.0. You can see more patients in the same time without compromising on the quality of cure.

3. Arrive at the Correct Remedy quickly. Use various filters to narrow down the choice of the remedy using your expertise.Filters like "Drug Filter" mineral, plant and Animal filter, intelligent Cilpboards to choose important symptoms, etc make your task of filtering drugs easy.

4. Get the Similimum - You can find the right remedy, right potency and right repetition using the Similimum function.Only Hompath offers you this unique benefit.

5. Get better results using the various strategies used by the Masters in Homeopathy like the Kentian method, Boenn method and Boger method.

6. You are able to record symptoms which are normaly not recorded by using the strong, fast and intelligent search which allows out to use Themes, Cross Refrences, Word Meanings, Similar, Vital and Essential words which widens your choice of symptoms.

7. Confirm the symptoms found in the repertory with the exact words of a prover or patient from the Materia Medica.

8. You can also refer your cases for a second opinion or present it in your meetings or seminars using the Pack and Go feature, which allows you to do so.

9. Understand Remedies and their inter-relationships by using the various features like Drug properties, Keynotes, Converting repertory to Materia medica and Group symptoms features.

10. Evaluate and understand your successes by using the Case Analysis module, which helps you to understand your cases in a graphical manner, as well as creating your own patient research.

11. Organise your appointments and schedules using the Hompath Assist module, which helps you, maintain a database of your contacts, manage your finances, print reports and certificates.

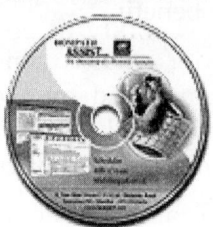

12. Keep in touch with the Global Homeopathic World with the Links Tresorie, a collection of articles from the Links International since 1987. Search by Author, Subject, Remedy, etc, from this unique collection.

13. Refer the Wisdom of last 200 years from the Tresorie, a collection of over 4000 articles from various renowned Journals.

14. You can access the Archives of over 300 Books in the Archives module, on various subjects like Materia Medica, Philosophy, Therapeutics, Clinical etc. Read and refer them at leisure.

15. Get complete details on Remedies from Materia Medica Elite and Materia Medica Live, which explain selected remedies in an interesting and easy to understand method using sounds and presentations.

16. Experience ease of operation and navigation. The Premium collection comes packed with a host of friendly tools, which can be accessed at one mouse click from a single screen.

HOMPATH WILDFIRE EXPERT SYSTEM SOFTWARE

Some feature of this software include:

- 35 repertories including Complete Repertory (2011 edition!)
- 270+Books of Materia Medica, Philosophy and Organon, Therapeutics, Regional Therapeutics, Clinical, Remedy picture and Pharmacy
- Very user-friendly software
- Quick Repertorization: Enter keywords of rubrics and Repertorize instantly, No need to know the symptom exactly as in repertory.
- Advance search to includes Synonyms and similar words
- Excellent Search speed and accuracy
- Drug filter makes selection of right medicine easy
- Simillimum: Guides to the selection of potency and repetition
- Expert Systems: Kentian, Boenninghausen and Boger's, True expert systems
- Cross references in repertory screen
- Themes: the concepts for selection of rubrics on general spoken words
- Family, Group, Subgroup analysis
- Group symptoms
- Trillions of Repertorisation analysis

- Keynotes, Drug relation, Drug properties, Open MM from Repertorisation itself
- Remedy comparison from Materia Medica with sections on a single screen
- Easy readability of books in HTML mode
- Interface of Repertory with Materia Medica
- Text to voice recognition to listen books
- User Manual of 425 pages with on-screen Help
- Patient Management system included
- Daily Auto-backup of patient data

You will also get:

o   197000 pages of information.
o   1000000 of symptoms in entire software.
o   5000+ cured cases.
o   3000 remedies and their information.
o   5000+ articles.
o   3187 clinical tips.
o   1000 volumes of data and books.
o   537 allopathic drug data.
o   4 expert systems.

The complete list of repertories in this special collection include:	
Complete Repertory	Roger Van Zandervoot
Repertory of Homoeopathic Materia Medica	Kent, J.T.
Therapeutic Pocket Book	Boenninghausen
Boenninghausen's Characteristics and Repertory	Boger, C.M.
Repertory to the symptoms of Intermittent fever	Allen, W.A
Index to Materia Medica	Allen
Boericke's repertory	Boericke, G.W.
Repertory of Herings Guiding symptoms of our Materia Medica	Knerr, C. B.
Synoptic Key	Boger, C.M.
Clinical Repertory	Clarke, J. H.
Concise repertory of Homoeopathy	Phatak, S.R.
Concordance Repertory of Materia Medica (6 Vols.)	Gentry, W.D.
Repertory to the more Characteristic Symptoms	Lippe, c.
Sensations as if.	Roberts, H.A.
Unabridged Dictionary of Sensations (Vol 2)	Ward, J.W.

This software will work on WINDOWS computers and MAC computers with Windows simulation.

III. RADAR (RAPID AID TO DRUG AIMED RESEARCH)

RADAR set the standard for homeopathy software, and now the best is even better. The arrival of **RADAR 10** brings major new features and a host of streamlined advances that take homeopathic software to a new level of excellence. The foundation of RADAR 10 is the new Synthesis 9.2 Repertory database. It's one of 20 repertories you can access with the program – along with the highly respected Complete 2003 and Repertorium Universale. And now you have the ability to search through all Repertories simultaneously. With RADAR 10, you can now find synonymous or related rubrics directly from the repertorization chart. Operations that required several screens in previous versions are now available to you from just one place, with a single click. You can even get immediate tool tip help with a simple touch of your mouse. In fact, the program now offers total integration between Clipboard and Analysis. And Analysis is even further expanded by the addition of Families, Miasmatic, Boenninghausen's Concordances and Relationship of Remedy functions.Using the Synthesis Repertory side by side with Roger van Zandvoort's Complete Millennium and Repertorium Universale is a dream come true. Now we have the freedom to compare and choose from all the available homoeopathic data.

Following are its features:

* **The Concepts Finder**

    Translate the language of your patient into the language of the Repertory. Use the Concepts Finder to add symptoms to your repertorization.

* **Radar Free Notes**

    Download the latest seminar notes, videos, ... Upload your personal notes to exchange with other homeopaths.

* **Live Update**

    Automaticaclly upgrades you, free of chanrge, to Radar program updates, Synthesis Update Logfiles, Free Notes, etc.

* **Improved Multimedia**

    200 new remedy pictures and 205 new sound clips. Visualize more remedies than ever before, listen to masters in homeopathy.

* **Improved families functions**

    Limit your analysis by selecting from different family groups or create your own groups.

* **Luc De Schepper module**

    Select the most important symptoms of your patient into the pyramid of Dr. Luc and differentiate remedies on the basis of the core delusion.

* **Ewald Stoeteler module**

    Offers a new method for homoeopathic analysis and practice, using Hahnemann's classification of diseases.

* **Two miasmatic approaches**

    The miasmatic analysis following Dr. Giampietro (Argentina) can be used with Radar 10 and Synthesis 9.2. Also, Sankaran's miasmatic database has been updated for optimal use within Radar 10.

* **Two new clinical files**

   Radar 10 links to KENBO and to HomeoPlus, 2 clinical practice management files.

* **Other miscellaneous improvements**

   Right mouse click on any remedy abbreviation in the repertory screen, now offers a choice of shortcuts, etc.

<u>16 other repertories detail:</u>

Boger, CM	–	Boenninghausen's Characteristics and Repertory
Boger, CM	–	Synoptic Key of the Materica Medica
Boger, CM	–	General Analysis
Boericke	–	Repertory in Pocket Manual
Clarke	–	Clinical Repertory
Ward	–	Sensations As If
Roberts	–	Sensations As If
Bhatia, VR	–	Miniature Repertory of Remedies in Common Cold
Choudhury	–	Hints for Treatment of Cancer
Drake, OM	–	Repertory of Warts and Condylomata
Foster	–	Toothache and its Cure
Jefferson Guernsey	–	Repertory of Hemorrhoids
Master, FJ	–	Hair Loss
Pulford, A and TD	–	Repertory of Pneumonia
Sudarshan, SR	–	Repertory of Non-Malarial evers
Sukumaran, N	–	Main Symptoms of Heart Problems

Radar Modules

- <u>Bönninghausen Method</u>
- <u>Concepts</u>
- <u>Families</u>
- <u>Giampietro</u>
- <u>Luc de Schepper Module</u>
- <u>The Kenbo Module</u>
- <u>Multimedia Features</u>
- <u>Sankaran Miasmatic</u>
- <u>Sherr Casetaker</u>
- <u>Vakil Module</u>
- <u>Vithoulkas Expert System</u>

IV. CARA

CARA PRO comes with a full fledged materia medica search engine already built in. This search engine, a program named Similia, was previously available only separately. Now it has become an integral part of CARA PRO and offers many classical as well as contemporary materia medica texts. As the second player in the multi media field, after RADAR, CARA PRO supports the display of color remedy images and playing of audio and video clips. David Witko claims that full color photographs of the remedies are included, but how many and of which quality remains to be seen. There will also be spoken text on some remedies by a few of the world's leading homeopaths.

Apart from that, CARA PRO will also offer a new repertory search method, which is by "theme". This sounds reminiscent of RADAR's semiological concepts. The appearance of rubric presentations has been improved, so that CARA PRO on screen looks like your familiar repertory book. In addition, it appears that several previous limitations of the program have been removed and enhanced.

Repertories

Standard repertories:

- Combined Repertory
- Homeopathic Medical Repertory (Robin Murphy)
- Boericke's Repertory
- Phatak's Repertory
- Boger-Boenninghausen's Repertory
- Clarke's Clinical Repertory

Optional repertory you can add:

- Complete Repertory (Roger van Zandvoort)

Materia Medicas

Standard books provided: 65 works in total:

- Hahnemann's Organon, Materia Medica Pura & Chronic Diseases
- Allen's Encyclopedia, Handbook & Keynotes
- Kent Lectures & Lesser Writings
- Boericke's Materia Medica
- Phatak's Materia Medica
- Anshutz New, Old & Forgotten Remedies
- Lilienthal Therapeutics
- Reversed Combined Repertory
- Clarke's Dictionary
- Lippe's Redline MM
- Boenninghausen Lesser Writings
- Cowperthwaite's Textbook
- Clarke's Prescriber and Collected Writings (20 books in all)
- Close Genius of Homeopathy
- Hughes Cyclopedia
- Burnett's Collected Writings (21 books in all)
- Farrington's Clinical MM, Lesser Writings & Therapeutic Pointers
- Roberts, Sensations As If

Optional books you can add:

- Vermeulen: Synoptic 1, Synoptic 2, Concordant

- Scholten: Minerals, Elements
- Sherr: Dynamic Provings
- Sankaran: Soul, Spirit, Substance, Provings, Elements
- Murphy: Lotus Materia Medica
- Mirilli: Thematic Materia Medica
- Verspoor: Homeopathy Renewed
- Boedler: Psychic Causes of Illness

Searching
- Search all repertories simultaneously for words
- Search all materia medicas simultaneously for words
- Search the repertory using theme words
- Browse the repertory
- Remedy addition author names displayed on screen (where appropriate)
- Compare up to 10 remedies across an entire repertory or selected chapters

Multimedia
- Hundreds of color remedy photographs
- Over 100 audio presentations from respected homeopathic teachers

Analysis
- Comprehensive remedy classification – by family, plant species, element, animal, nosode, insect, snake and so on
- Analysis by Family of remedy, Miasm, Species and Periodic Table
- Emphasise rubrics
- 36 different repertorisation strategies
- Contains a sophisticated Expert System to help analyse your cases

General
- Patient record database
- Record a visit for each consultation
- Make your own additions to the repertory
- Annotate any rubric or materia medica
- Create new rubrics from materia medica searches
- Combine up to 10 rubrics to form new rubrics for analysis

System Requirements
- PC running Windows 95/98/NT
- Minimum 16 Mb RAM, 32 Mb recommended
- CD-ROM drive
- 256 colour screen or better
- Minimum disk space 120Mb
- Full system requires 776Mb available disk space
- Cara will also run on Apple Mac computers using the Real PC emulator.

V. STIMULARE

A case taking and Repertorisation software developed by Qu - Bit Homoeo technologies, Bangalore is a highly helpful tool to all homeopaths. With its powerful features and affordable pricing it is emerging as one of the best alternatives to current market leaders.

Stimulare has two sections in it.

1) The most appealing one is the Case sheet.

2) The other section is the one with powerful repertories in it.

1) The case sheet.

This case sheet is developed with individuality of homeopaths in mind. A section of homeopaths always like to type in their case and this case sheet allow you to do exactly that in all the sections. Type in as much information as you like. In the end after you decide on the remedy and type it in just save and close. It will not restrict you to any one mode during the case taking. If you wish to enter data in one section by typing and another section by selection from an available list you can do that too.

If you are of the second type you can enter the entire case data by selecting from the list in each section. Just double click against the heading and select from the list.

During the process of case taking itself you can add the symptoms/Rubrics and by the time you finish of you can repertorise at the click of a button and get to the right remedy.

The unique feature of this software is that it allows you to create your very own suggestions and database by editing the 'masters' to suit your requirement. You need not want to run to the manufacturer each time you need minor additions.

It also allows you to add your clinic information entered and saved so that whenever you take a print out this field can be put in it.

The case taking section allows you to get print outs which are neat and compact. You can select the fields to get printed.

The case can be copied and pasted to MS Word or your email editor and sent as email to seek suggestions and opinions on the case if you are in the habit of doing so.

The case sheet also allows you to do statistical analysis of your cases on the basis of various features.

The biggest draw back that I found is that it will not allow you to underline or color code significant points while taking the case. But Qu - Bit says it is working on the matter.

2) The second section deals with repertory.

There are three different versions of Stimulare.

A) The Basic version has Such powerful repertories as Kent, Boenninghausen, Boger, Pathak etc.

B) The Professional version has in addition Complete repertory [basic].

C) The Complete version can boast of Complete repertory 2005 and Universalis repertory 2005.

The repertories open in such a way that the left side window list the repertories and chapters while the right one has the rubrics.

Four levels of search and selection are available. A unique feature of the search is that it allows simultaneous two word search. With the books and chapters opening sided by side with the main window the busy practitioner is saved of much time since it allows easy migration between various repertories and chapters of the same repertory.

Advantages:

1) The unique feature of this software is that it allows you to create your very own suggestions and database by editing the 'masters' to suit your requirement. You need not want to run to the manufacturer each time you need minor addition

2) It also allows you to add your clinic information entered and saved so that whenever you take a print out this field can be put in it.

3) The case taking section allows you to get print outs which are neat and compact. You can select the fields to get printed.

4) The case can be copied and pasted to MS Word or your email editor and sent as email to seek suggestions and opinions on the case if you are in the habit of doing so.

5) The case sheet also allows you to do statistical analysis of your cases on the basis of various features.

Drawback :

1) The biggest draw back that I found is that it will not allow you to underline or color code significant points while taking the case.

VI. ISIS

The latest version of Miccant's ISIS system, ISIS Vision answers the need for increased ease of use and more powerful and sophisticated repertory and materia medica searching. Offering all of the convenience and practicality of ISIS, but with added speed, power and flexibility, ISIS Vision is still the only software of its kind to combine repertories, materia medicas, remedy database, dictionaries and more in one convenient and simple interface. The result is incredible ease of use! The only draw back is that it doesn't contains synthetic repertory. They are offering free up gradation.

VII. ORGANON 1996

It is based on the SCR system in use at I.C.R Bombay. Dr.M.L.Dhawale systematized homoeopathy by integrating the approaches of Boger, Boenninghausen and Kent. Based on a sound integral clinical experience, there is a live demonstration of first six aphorismsof "Organon of Medicine" in SCR system.This is a user friendly programme which attempts to incorporate these hence the name " ORGANON 96".

Version 2.1 of the Homeopathy Program ORGANON 2001 has been released and is now available in two editions: the Basic and the Advanced edition.A major advantage of this program is that it is time effective. The ADVANCED version includes 3,592,918 references to medicines, approximately 2,700,000 references to medicines, which are based on synthetic thinking and concern compounds of two or three chemical elements, are presented to homeopaths around the world for the first time.The program functions are very simple, comprehensible and user-friendly, even for the most inexperienced computer users. The entire symptom search process is completed on one screen where all necessary information appears simultaneously, Information available in 28 languages.

BIBLIOGRAPHY

1) Barthel,H and Will K, Synthetic Repertory, New Delhi. Indian reprint (B.Jain)

2) Bidwell, Glen Irving, How to use a Repertory, New Delhi, Indian reprint (B.Jain)

3) Boenninghausen, C.Von, A Systematic, Alphabetic Repertory of Homoeopathic Remedies, New Delhi, Indian reprint (B.Jain)

4) Boericke William, Pocket Manual Of Homoeopathic Materia Medica with Repertory, New Delhi, Indian reprint (B.Jain)

5) Boericke Grath, Principles of Homoeopathy, New Delhi, Indian reprint (B.Jain)

6) Boger .C.M. Addition to Kent's Repertory, New Delhi, Indian reprint (B.Jain)

   Boennighausen's Characteristics and Repertory, New Delhi, Indian reprint (B.Jain)

   General Analysis, Seventh Edition, Bombay, 1959 (Roy & Co.)

   Studies in Philosophies and Healing, Second Edition, Bombay 1964, (Roy & Co.)

   Synoptic Key of the Materia Medica, New Delhi, Indian reprint (B.Jain)

7) Bradford, Thomas Lindsley, Lesser Writings of C.M.F.Von Boenninghausen, New Delhi, Indian reprint (B.Jain)

8) Castro, J. Benedict, Encyclopaedia of Repertory, New Delhi, Indian reprint (B.Jain)

9) Chris Kruz, Computer Repertories, A comparison, Resource Homoeopathy, Sep/Oct. Vol.19, Number-5

10) Clarke, J.H, A Clinical Repertory to the Dictionary of Materia Medica, New Delhi, Indian reprint (B.Jain)

11) Dhawale, M.L., Principles and Practice of Homoeopathy. Vol.I, Homoeopathic Philosophy and Repertorisation, Second Edition, Bombay, 1985(Institute for Clinical Research)

    Symposium, Area C & D, Bombay, 1978

12) Gentry, William .D., Concordance Repertory of More Characteristic Symptoms of Materia Medica, New Delhi, Indian reprint (B.Jain)

13) Gypser,K.H, Kent's Minor Writings on Homoeopathy, New Delhi, Indian reprint (B.Jain)

14) Hael, Richard, Samuel Hahnemann, His Life & Work, Vols. I & II, New Delhi, Indian reprint (B.Jain)

15) Hahnemann, S.C.F., Organon Of Medicine, Sixth Edition, New Delhi, Indian reprint (B.Jain)

    Materia Medica Pura, New Delhi, Indian reprint (B.Jain)

16) Harinadham, K., The Principles and Practice of Repertorization, Indian Books & Periodicals Publishers, New Delhi, 2002

17) Isselbacher, Harrison's Principles of Internal Medicine, Mc Graw Hill, Inc, New York, Thirteenth Edition 1994.

18) Farrrington, Harvey, Homoeopathy & Homoeopathic Prescribing, New Delhi, Indian reprint (B.Jain)

19) Jawahar Shah- Dr. Homoeopathic Classic, Users Guide, 10/11 Harish Kunj, 16 , Tagore Road, Santacruz (West) Mumbai-54

20) Kanjilal, J.N., Repertorization, Second Edition, New Delhi, 1984, (B.Jain)

21) Kent, J.T., Lectures on Homoeopathic Materia Medica, New Delhi, Indian reprint (B.Jain)

Lectures on Homoeopathic Philosophy, New Delhi, Indian reprint (B.Jain)

Repertory of Homoeopathic Materia Medica, New Delhi, Indian reprint (B.Jain)

Use of Repertory: How to study the repertory, How to use the repertory, New Delhi, Indian reprint (B.Jain)

What the Doctor Needs to know in order to make a successful prescription, New Delhi, Indian reprint (B.Jain)

22) Kishor, Jugal, Index to Card Repertory, New Delhi, 1959

23) Kishor, Jugal, evolution of Homoeopathic Repertories and Repertorisation, Kishor Card Publication, New Delhi, 1998

24) Knerr, Calvin B., Repertory of Hering's Guiding Symptoms of our Materia Medica, New Delhi, Indian reprint (B.Jain)

25) Lippe, Constantine, Repertory to more Characteristics Symptoms of Materia Medica, New Delhi, Indian reprint (B.Jain)

26) Master, Jamshed Farokh, Percieving Rubrics of the Mind, New Delhi, 1989 (B..Jain)

27) Robin Murphy, Homoeopathic Medical Repertory, Indian Books and Periodicals syndicate, New Delhi, First edition , 1994

28) Patel. R.P., Art of Case taking and Practical Repertorization, Fourth edition, Kottayam, , 1986

29) Roberts.H.A, Boenninghausen's Therapeutic Pocket Book, New Delhi, Indian reprint (B.Jain)

30) Roberts.H.A , Sensations As If ......, New Delhi, Indian reprint (B.Jain)

31) Sarkar.B.K, Essentials of Homoeopathic Philosophy and Place of Repertory in Homoeopathic practice, Calcutta, 1955 [M.Bhattacharya & Co.]

32) Schroyens Fredricke, Synthesis, Homoeopathic Book Publishers London, B.Jain Publishers, New Delhi, 1993 , Edition 7.2

33) Stedman- Stedman's Medical Dictionary, Williams & Wilkins, Baltimore 26 th edition, 1995

34) Stimulare –2014-2015, User Manual Homoeopathic Software, Qu- Bit Homoeo Technologies, No-20, Banglore University Layout, BEML 5th stage park, Raja Rajeshwari , Banglore.

35) Tarafdar, D., Repertory Explained, Calcutta 1986[Modern Homoeopathic Publications]

36) Tiwari, Shashi Kant, Essentials of Repertorisation, B. Jain Publishers, New Delhi, Fourth edition, 2005.

37) Tiwari, Shashi Kant, Homoeopathy and Child Care, B. Jain Publishers, New Delhi, First Edition, 1998

38) Tyler, M.L. Homoeopathic Drug Picture, New Delhi, Indian reprint (B. Jain)

39) Tyler M.l. and John, Weir, Repertorising, New Delhi, Indian reprint (B.Jain).

40) Vithoulkas, George, Additions to Kents Repertory, New Delhi, 1989 (B.Jain)

41) Wright, Elizabeth, A Breif Study Course in Homoeopathy, New Delhi, Indian reprint (B. Jain)

42) W.B. Saunders Dictionary Staff- Dorland's Illustrated Medical Dictionary, W.B. Saunders Company, Philadelphia, 28 th Edition 1994